T5-DHU-038

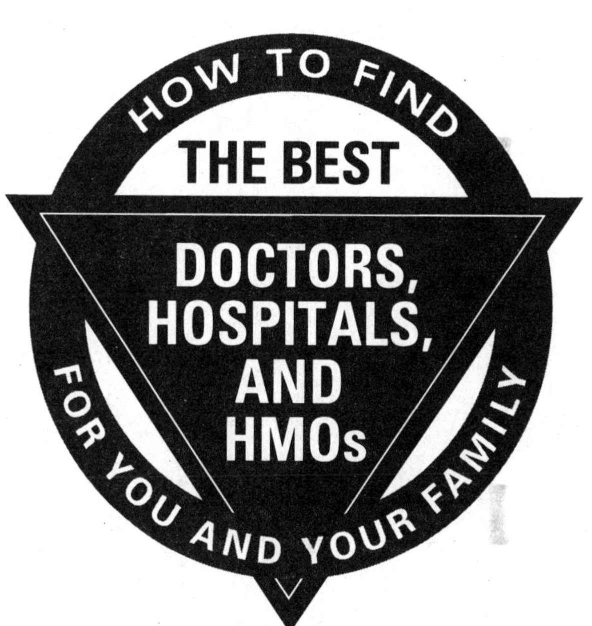
HOW TO FIND
THE BEST
DOCTORS,
HOSPITALS,
AND
HMOs
FOR YOU AND YOUR FAMILY

CASTLE CONNOLLY

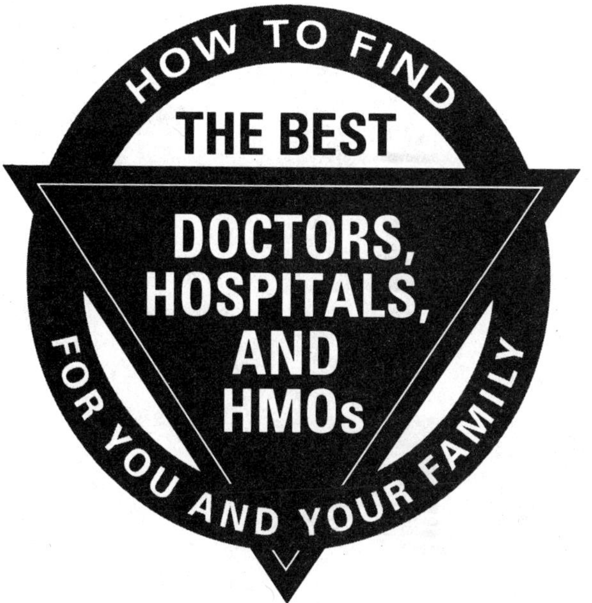

POCKET GUIDE

Castle Connolly Medical Ltd.
New York

Castle Connolly Pocket Guide: How To Find the Best Doctors, Hospitals, and HMOs for You and Your Family

Library of Congress Catalog Card Number 94-92449

The purpose of the book is educational and informational. It is not intended to replace the advice of your physician or to assist the layman in diagnosing or treating illness, disease or injury. Following the advice or recommendations set forth in this book is entirely at the reader's own risk. The author and publishers cannot ensure accuracy of, or assume responsibility for, the information in the book as such information is affected by constant change.

ISBN 1-883769-70-1

PRINTED IN THE UNITED STATES OF AMERICA

"I spend more time choosing a good bottle of wine than a hospital or physician."

— Arthur Miller

Harvard Professor of Law and TV personality, commenting at an American Hospital Association annual meeting.

Acknowledgments

The publishers wish to thank the many people who lent their time, creative thoughts, expertise, and effort to this undertaking.

We are grateful to the many physicians and other health professionals who offered advice, criticism, editorial comments, and encouragement throughout the process. Of course, a special thanks goes to those staff, editors, research assistants, and our publications coordinator who worked tirelessly as a team to complete this book.

Table of Contents

Section Four
Cost, Quality, and Consumers: You Can Cut Your Health Care Costs. Here's How.

Section Five
Special Health Care Choices: Consider the Needs of Women, Children, Older Adults, and Emergency Patients. Here's How.

Section Six
Appendixes

Foreword

Paul M. Ellwood, MD,
Chairman, Jackson Hole Group

Unlike many responsibilities we take on—raising our children, planning for retirement, or buying a house—there are few resources to prepare us for finding and purchasing medical care. Most consumers have learned what they know about the health care system from their own experiences or the experiences of their friends and families. The authors of this book have taken a bold step in revealing the inner workings of the US health care system. They have provided a valuable map to physician office practices, indemnity health insurance, hospitals, and HMOs. Unfortunately, many who reach for this book in time of illness will find that some of the most important decisions that will affect their care will have already been made.

Health care is different from other things we buy. In most cases we can't afford to pay for expensive health care out of our own pockets, so we purchase insurance to pay our unplanned medical bills. Although premiums change, they are more predictable than the costs of medical care, especially in the event of serious illness. To further com-

plicate this purchase, most of us have premiums taken out of our paychecks and that distances us even farther from the real cost of medical care.

Because it would be best to make decisions about what kind of health care we want while we are healthy and don't have immediate medical need, it would pay us all to read this book and think through our health care purchasing decisions before we get sick.

Great changes are underway in the US health care system. Whether or not there are new laws at the federal or state level, the health care system is reorganizing itself and you, as a consumer of health care, are the reason for these changes. Individual consumers and organized purchasers, such as employers, have demanded that costs come down and that patients receive effective, appropriate treatment.

In a sense, you are the driver of reform. I would like to give you a few things to think about as you read this book and make health care choices for yourself and your family.

- *You cannot evaluate health care on the basis of cost alone. Look for providers who can demonstrate that they provide good care. Beware of providers who make broad, sweeping statements about a commitment to quality and look closely at providers who are measuring the results of their care. These measures, referred to as outcomes, are not based on activities like how many treatments were done, but on how well the patients did as a result of the treatment.*

- *Many organizations are just beginning to measure outcomes. Because the field of outcome measurement is so new, the authors of this book also have described traditional ways of evaluating quality so you can understand the credentials and reports you will find most often. But, when you have the chance, ask for records that are based on patient reports and ratings rather than organizational audits or test results. For instance, a health plan or physicians' practice that tracks how diabetic patients rate the ways their condition affects their daily life gives you more information than being told the number of diabetics who receive an eye exam each year.*

- *More care is not necessarily better care, since unnecessary procedures result not only in waste, but often in worse health status. This is especially true of invasive procedures. Recent studies have found that patients who have surgery for benign prostrate problems often develop complications that are worse than the condition.*

Let me leave you with a simple description of what the health care system, and the people who comprise it, should do for you. It should encourage and help you to achieve the physical and emotional health you need for daily life, it should limit the ravages of disease as well as current medicine can, and it should prevent avoidable disease and death. I hope this book is a valuable guide in your search for health care for you and your family.

Paul M. Ellwood, MD
Jackson Hole, WY

A Letter from Louis W. Sullivan, MD

**A Letter from Louis W. Sullivan, MD
President, Morehouse School of Medicine
and former Secretary of Health and
Human Services**

The issue of health care is one that has been increasingly prominent in the nation's consciousness in recent years. It is a troubling issue—and a troubling time—for many Americans.

The lack of health insurance for many is only one concern. We ponder questions of quality and we are concerned about possible limits on choice. And while we recognize the shortcomings of our system, we want our nation's leaders to proceed carefully, lest we do more harm than good in seeking the solutions to our problems.

As Americans, our relationship with health care providers often has been an uncertain and changing one. Medical practice has evolved from the period of the general practitioner to the age of the specialist. Hospitals have grown increasingly complex, with the concept of the "medical center" rather than hospital as the predominant one in many communities. Managed care, only a few decades ago a pioneering concept born on the west coast, is now a major presence in health care delivery throughout the nation.

Throughout this change, and our difficulty at times in adjusting to it, major achievements have marked our progress. Many childhood diseases have been all but eliminated; new diagnostic technology and drugs have been introduced; therapies envisioned only in laboratories are now readily available at the bedside; and a greater emphasis on prevention and wellness has taken hold in the health professions as well as with the public .

However, much remains to be done. Reforming our health care system is not going to happen in a day. It is a process now occurring wherever there are patients in need, caring providers, and the organizational systems and financial support to ensure the delivery of care.

During the years of change that lie ahead, we need to become "informed, assertive consumers." We need to take responsibility for our own health and be prepared to make difficult choices, not only of doctors, hospitals, and health plans, but of legislative proposals and reform initiatives. To do this effectively—to understand and make wise choices—we will need tools like the Castle Connolly Pocket Guide.

To the readers, I wish good health and to the publishers, I wish success.

Sincerely,

Louis W. Sullivan, MD

Preface

The problem of where to find the best health care is one that most people face on a fairly regular basis.

During any given year a typical family may be cared for by a number of doctors: an internist for male or female adults; a gynecologist for female adults; a pediatrician for children; an ophthalmologist; a dermatologist; a psychiatrist; an orthopedist, or perhaps a general surgeon. At the same time, family members may also face hospitalization on a few occasions over a period of years. And, with more and more Americans choosing managed care every year, selecting from HMOs and other managed care programs is a challenge many of us will face.

As Chairman of the Board of New York Medical College, and as a Commissioner of the Joint Commission on Accreditation of Healthcare Organizations, John Castle was often called by friends or associates for recommendations of doctors and hospitals. He naturally turned to John J. Connolly, the President of New York Medical College, for his suggestions. Castle reasoned that if his friends and associates had such a difficult time finding the right health care providers, others would as well, and he suggested to Dr. Connolly that they publish a book to help people make these difficult but critical choices. Thus, the concept of this guide was born.

Health care reform will not solve the dilemma of who to select to provide health care. President Clinton has promised that under any reform, Americans will be able to choose their own doctors. And clearly, with managed care playing an increasing role in most health care delivery systems, Americans will need to know how to select from the variety of plans offered, as well as how to make wise choices of doctors and hospitals within plans. Managed care limits choices, and that makes choosing wisely even more important. The Castle Connolly Pocket Guide: How to Find the Best Doctors, Hospitals, and HMOs for You and Your Family *will help you make these important choices in an informed fashion. With the* Castle Connolly Pocket Guide *as a reference, you will know what criteria to look for, what information to seek, where to find it, and how to understand and use it.*

The Castle Connolly Pocket Guide *was written with the assistance of doctors, health care experts, hospital and HMO executives, and consumers. We hope that it will be a significant aid in helping you find the best health care for you and your family.*

Introduction

How this Book Can Help You Improve Your Health

A savvy consumer, searching for a car, restaurant, house, or even a spouse, can easily find a guidebook to help. Yet, when it comes to choosing health care providers, the bookshelves are nearly bare.

The *Castle Connolly Pocket Guide: How to Find the Best Doctors, Hospitals, and HMOs for You and Your Family* has been written to fill that void. It will guide you in making critical—even lifesaving—choices.

This book has two goals:

1. To provide you with a base of information and a framework of understanding so that you can select the best doctors, hospitals, and HMOs to meet your health care needs and those of your family.

2. To identify and explain a variety of useful resources and specific health-related information that you can use to improve your health care and that of your family.

Medicine is often described as a combination of art and science. This description holds true for the process of selecting the best medical care. This book describes the "science" of making that selection. It is not magical or even difficult. It is simply a matter of knowing what information you should have and where to find it.

The "art" is what you will bring to the selection process. It is based upon your feelings, your needs, and the chemistry that develops between you and those who provide your health care. The *Castle Connolly Pocket Guide* will help you prepare for that interaction and guide you in getting the most from it.

Most important, The *Castle Connolly Pocket Guide: How to Find the Best Doctors, Hospitals, and HMOs* will tell you how to combine the art and science so that you can make the best choices.

How to Use this Book

This book has been written as a basic, "how to" guide to selecting the best health care. Each of the five sections in the book addresses a specific area of health care. Each chapter contains important background information on a single aspect of the area.

There are two effective ways to use this book:

1. Read it cover to cover. This method will give you a broad understanding of the health care field and a clearer perspective of where you fit into it.

2. Select certain chapters from the Table of Contents to study for specific information. This method will arm you with information necessary to make immediate choices.

   At the beginning of each section is a list of explanations of terms that may be new to you. Reviewing this list will help you read the section easily.

   In the final section are 16 appendixes. Together these listings contain more than 250 sources for getting help on virtually any question you might have about health and health care. In addition, you will find detailed descriptions of the information on doctors, hospitals, and HMOs that state health departments will release to consumers.

Finally, at the back of the book you will find a postage paid return card. We want to hear what you think of the *Castle Connolly Pocket Guide* and how we can improve it to meet your needs. We will also alert you to the publication of a *Castle Connolly Regional Guide* for your area. It will list doctors we have carefully screened and describe the hospitals and HMOs in your community.

Section One

The Doctor of Choice: Choosing a Doctor Calls for Savvy Consumerism. Read on.

Key Terms

▼ **American Board of Medical Specialties (ABMS)**

The organization that oversees and coordinates the 24 medical specialty boards that approve residency programs in 25 specialties and govern standards within each specialty.

▼ **Clinical**

A term referring to direct contact with, or information from, patients.

▼ **Efficacy**

The effectiveness or ability of a drug or treatment to bring about the desired results.

▼ **Generic**

Pertains to drugs that are not of name brand. Doctors may often prescribe the less expensive, generic versions of brand-name drugs.

▼ **Health Maintenance Organization (HMO)**

A managed care organization that provides for a wide range of comprehensive health care services for its members for a fixed, predetermined fee. The care is provided by a closed panel of physicians and possibly other health care professionals.

▼ Indemnity Plan

Health insurance plan that pays a predetermined dollar amount for a specific type of care; for example, $50 for an office visit to a doctor. The patient typically pays the difference, if any, between the charge and the reimbursed fee.

▼ Lupus Erythematosus

An autoimmune disorder characterized by inflammation. Usually involving several organ systems, lupus erythematosus most commonly manifests itself by skin lesions and joint pain as well as decreased cell counts.

▼ Lyme Disease

Named for Lyme, Connecticut, where it was first identified, Lyme disease is transmitted through the bite of a deer tick that may or may not produce a distinctive "bull's-eye" rash. Other symptoms may include flu-like aches, arthritic joint pain, and, in complicated cases, cardiac abnormalities.

▼ Managed Care

The process of integrating the finance and delivery of health care to control costs and improve quality. A managed care plan typically involves a group of practitioners who "manage" care for a specified population.

▼ Specialist

A physician who practices one or more of the 25 specialties defined by the American Board of Medical Specialties (ABMS). Also, a general term used to describe a doctor's general area of practice (surgery, pediatrics, etc.).

▼ Subspecialist

A physician, already board-certified, who has obtained further training and certification in one or more medical specialties of the 50 subspecialty certifications offered by the American Board of Medical Specialties (ABMS).

Primary Care Physicians: Doctors Who See You Through Sickness and Health

Chapter 1

When it comes to choosing a doctor, most people let the decision slide until they are sick or hurt and need medical attention fast. That's unfortunate if an illness that could have been managed successfully develops to a stage where it becomes difficult to control or cure. It's even more unfortunate if the illness could have been prevented in the first place.

The time to establish a relationship with a doctor is *while you are healthy*. And the doctor to establish your relationship with is the one who is most likely to keep you healthy: a primary care physician.

Primary means first, so a primary care doctor is the first one you see for any health problem. Primary also means basic, so a primary care doctor offers the kind of fundamental care that can keep you healthy.

Yes, You *Do* Need a Doctor When You're Healthy.

Here are four good reasons why you should start your search for a primary care doctor now:

Reason One

A primary care doctor can put your medical condition in context. It is difficult for any doctor, however skilled, to make judgements based on only one visit or a single test. Conditions well out of normal range are easy to pick up, but extreme variations do not always occur, and a serious illness may develop slowly with only a gradual increase in symptoms. The operative word is continuity: ideally, your medical care should not be interrupted by changes in providers.

Reason Two

A primary care doctor is better able to treat you as a whole person. Medicine has become very specialized and procedure-oriented, but the human body is not a loose collection of unrelated parts. It is a "whole," with strong interrelationships between all biological systems. And context is important: this consists of your medical history, current condition as compared with past medical status, and changes in your body and environment over time. Some of the poorest medical care results from people jumping from subspecialist to subspecialist. Despite talent, skill, and training, no specialist knows the patient well enough, or for long enough, to be able to take the whole person into consideration and track the normal patterns of evolution and change. We end up with a specialist for every organ and system instead of a doctor who will care for the whole person.

Our health care system does not place enough emphasis on preventing illness; most health care dollars are spent on curative, rather than preventive, medicine.

Reason Three

A primary care doctor can establish preventive programs. Our health care system does not place enough emphasis on preventing illness; most health care dollars are spent on curative, rather than preventive, medicine. But the status quo is slowly changing, and it is within primary care that the change is most evident. Your primary care doctor can educate you about the hows and whys of health maintenance and disease prevention and follow up to help you stay faithful to the course the two of you have agreed upon. Only an ongoing relationship makes this possible.

Reason Four

A primary care doctor can save you money. Managed care advocates, among others, have long deplored the waste inherent in a system in which patients can simply call any specialist any time they have an ache or pain or are not feeling well. Primary care doctors can monitor referrals to specialists, following the patient closely to put together a variety of observations, opinions, and test results in order to treat each person on an individual basis. This improves the quality of care and also controls costs.

▼

A businessman in his late fifties, a long-time competitive runner, had surgery in one of St. Louis' top hospitals to repair a badly torn Achilles tendon. At his first follow-up visit to the orthopedic surgeon, he was assured that "everything was healing perfectly," that he had nothing to be concerned about, and that he would soon be up and running again. Shortly thereafter, just before a summer camping trip, he decided to have his yearly physical examination. The primary care doctor examined the site of the surgery, probing up and down the whole length of the leg. Explaining that he was concerned about certain swelling and discoloration, the doctor arranged for a further examination with ultrasound imaging. This sophisticated test showed that a blood clot had formed in the upper part of the leg, which could have caused severe disability and even death had it gotten into the bloodstream and traveled to the heart or brain. It was the primary care doctor, carefully conducting a full physical exam and who knew the patient well, who discovered the potentially fatal condition.

▼

Patients who visit specialists without some guidance from a primary care doctor may choose the wrong specialist based on a general observation and self-diagnosis about the problem or illness they're experiencing. While in some cases the problem may be obvious (for example, an eye injury), in others it may be more subtle. Diseases such as lupus erythematosus and Lyme disease, for example, often have myriad symptoms that are easily misinterpreted by laypersons; in fact, they are often difficult even for doctors to diagnose accurately. While certain problems may require the collaboration of several specialists, it is important to have a primary care doctor navigating the course.

There are five possible avenues to begin the process of finding a doctor that best suits your needs.

- *Doctor Referrals*
- *Friends and Relatives*
- *Hospital Referral Services*
- *Medical Society Directories*
- *Advertising*

Finally, it is estimated that almost half of all emergency room visits in some areas are for non-emergencies, an expensive and wasteful practice. When people have primary care doctors, they tend to turn to them rather than to hospital emergency departments.

If you are enrolled in any kind of managed care program, health maintenance organization (HMO) or other, you will almost always be required to select a primary care doctor from its roster. Managed care executives recognize the necessity of a primary care doctor, not only for delivering quality health care, but also for controlling costs.

How to Find a Doctor

Unless you already have a primary care doctor you are satisfied with, you will have to find one. How? Here are five possible avenues to begin the process of finding the doctor that best suits your needs. Each has limits, however.

Doctor Referrals

If you are moving and are leaving a trusted doctor behind, get a recommendation or two before you go. Furthermore, ask in what context and how well your doctor knows the new doctor—they may not have met since medical school.

Friends and Relatives

Always keep in mind that such recommendations are based largely on what may be "simpatico," or a personal affinity. Ask why your friend likes the doctor. It might be because the fees are low or the doctor makes house calls or is warm and sociable—all valid considerations, but certainly not principal determinants. So be wary of the generalized recommendation that "Dr. Jones is just wonderful." When considering recommendations, use the old navigational technique of triangulation: that is, focus on doctors whose names are mentioned by three or more people.

▼

One woman—a long-time Philadelphia resident who moved to a small town in Indiana to be near her children—found out the hard way about advice when she selected a doctor on the basis of her neighbor's glowing praise. During the initial visit, the patient's numerous questions about her chronic arthritis condition went unanswered while the doctor merely patted her on the shoulder and assured her that he "would take care of everything." While the paternalistic attitude might have suited the neighbor's needs, it fell far short for this senior patient, who was used to a good give-and-take with her former internist in Philadelphia. She resumed her search for a doctor—this time with the advice of her former doctor.

▼

Hospital Referral Services

Hospital telephone referral lines are not designed to distinguish among hundreds of doctors who may be more or less well regarded by other doctors, or who may be better suited to a particular caller when factors other than location, insurance coverage, and office hours are taken into consideration. It would be impolitic for hospital referral services to rate their members. Their recommendations are based on specialty and geographic proximity, usually by way of a computer that rotates through the lists to "recommend" the next three names in line, and all members of the medical staff are eligible to participate.

Medical Society Directories

Many local medical societies publish directories, some of which are intended primarily for doctor-to-doctor referrals, while others are distributed to the public. These directories usually provide names, addresses, phone numbers, and specialties, and can be useful sources. However, they do not distinguish among doctors in any way. All members of the medical society, usually a countywide organization, are eligible for inclusion. This also applies to the referral lines offered by many medical societies.

Advertising

> ***Tip***
>
> *Be aware that many referral lines accept any doctor who pays to be listed.*

Responding to advertising is the least effective way to find a doctor. While more and more health professionals now advertise, a practice which is no longer considered unethical, some stigma still remains. Advertising could lead you to a doctor who receives few or no referrals from colleagues and whose orientation to the profession is more entrepreneurial than medical. Most referral lines not sponsored by hospitals charge a fee to doctors who want to be listed. This is simply another form of advertising.

Many Ways to Say Doctor

In this book, the term "doctor" is used to describe only medical doctors who have received a doctor of medicine degree (MD) and osteopaths who have received a doctor of osteopathic medicine degree (DO). Doctors who have been trained in the British system may hold a degree of bachelor of medicine (MB), bachelor of surgery (BS), or bachelor of chirugia (BCh), which is based on the ancient Greek term that refers to surgery.

The more formal term for any of these practitioners is "physician." However, most people use the more popular term "doctor," which is the one generally used in this book. Our discussions do not include other kinds of doctors such as dentists or podiatrists or psychologists, who also deliver health care.

Primary Care: The Fundamental Four

There is not complete agreement in medicine on which specialties are practiced by the group of doctors known as primary care specialists. For the purposes of this book, we have included the following specialties: Internal Medicine; Pediatrics; Family Practice, and Obstetrics and Gynecology. Most adults choose specialists in internal medicine as their primary care doctors, and select pediatricians for their children. There is also a relatively new type of specialist, the family practitioner, who cares for both children and adults. In addition to such generalists, many women also select obstetrician/gynecologists as primary care providers.

A General Internist, *specializing in internal medicine, is trained to treat all internal organs and systems of the body. Many internists are also board-certified in a subspecialty, such as cardiology, gastroenterology, or geriatric medicine. Therefore, if you have a history of heart disease, you many wish to select an internist who has additional training in cardiology, but who primarily practices general internal medicine. On the other hand, your primary care doctor may refer you to a cardiologist when necessary, and both may treat you over a period of years. In fact, it is not unusual for a patient with a serious or complex illness to be followed by two or three doctors, with the primary care doctor "quarterbacking" the team.*

A study by the American College of Obstetrics and Gynecology showed that 54 percent of women who see a gynecologist use these doctors for primary care.

A Family Practitioner *belongs to a relatively new specialty. Such doctors come closest to the general practitioner of the past. They are qualified to treat all family members, including children.*

A Pediatrician *is the doctor you would choose for the care of your children. As with doctors in internal medicine, pediatricians often have a subspecialty such as cardiology, allergy and immunology, or endocrinology.*

Obstetricians and Gynecologists *are the subject of significant debate in terms of their appropriateness as primary care doctors. The American*

Board of Obstetrics and Gynecology states that these doctors are specialists and are not generally trained for primary care. However, the reality is that many, particularly those who solely practice gynecology, often serve as a woman's primary care doctor. Gynecologists are divided on the issue. One recent study showed that 95 percent of visits to ob-gyns are self-referred and that about 60 percent of visits to these specialists are for diagnostic services and preventive services. Another study, by the American College of Obstetrics and Gynecology, showed that 54 percent of women who see a gynecologist use these doctors for primary care. Reflecting the reality of current medical practice, we have included these specialists in the primary care category.

What Makes a Doctor "Best"?

Chapter 2

While the overwhelming majority of doctors are competent practitioners, some are less well trained or, for various other reasons, lack a desired level of professional skill or personal characteristics. They have met certain minimum standards, passed the necessary exams, and are licensed, but you would still be better off to avoid them. At the same time, among the many good doctors you could choose from, there will be some who are better for you and your family for a variety of reasons.

It is almost impossible to identify "the best" doctors in a particular specialty. There may be some who are generally acknowledged as leaders in a particular field, but that level of national reputation is typically built on appointments to important academic positions, innovative research, or the development of cutting-edge clinical techniques and treatments. Unless you are in need of those techniques and treatments, those doctors may not be the best for you. Since most people will obtain all, or certainly most, of their medical care near where they live, it is important for you to identify which doctors are among the best in your own community.

We do not argue that any single group of specialists is better than another as primary care doctors. You may have personal preferences based on criteria other than specialty, such as hospital affiliation, office location, practice characteristics, or personal traits, and that is how your selection should be made.

There are four broad areas of characteristics you should consider in selecting a primary care doctor:

- *Professional preparation, including education, residency training, board certification, and fellowships.*
- *Professional reputation.*
- *Office and practice arrangements.*
- *Professional (or bedside) manner.*

Professional Preparation

Education

Your review of your prospective doctor's education and training should begin with medical school. While you may feel that the institution where someone earned a bachelor's degree could be an indication of the quality of the doctor, most people in the medical field do not believe it plays a major role. A degree from a highly selective undergraduate college or university will help an aspiring doctor gain admission to a medical school, but once there, all students are peers. However, the information on undergraduate colleges, if important to you, is available in the American Board of Medical Specialties' (ABMS) *Compendium of Certified Medical Specialists* and other medical directories.

American medical schools are highly standardized, at least in terms of minimum quality. All US medical schools that grant medical degrees (MDs) and osteopathic degrees (DOs) are accredited by a group known as the LCME (Liaison Committee for Medical Education). Most are also accredited by the appropriate state agency, if one exists, and by regional accrediting agencies that accredit colleges and universities of all kinds.

Furthermore, US medical schools have universally high standards for admission, including success on the undergraduate level and on the Medical College Admissions Tests (MCATs). Although frequently criticized for being slow to change and for training too many specialists, the system of medical education in the United States has insured high quality in medical practice. One recent positive change is a strong effort in most medical schools to diversify the composition of the student body. While these schools have been less successful in enrolling racial minorities, the number of women has increased to the point that they now make up about 40 percent of most classes. In certain specialties preferred by women medical graduates (pediatrics, for example), it is possible that in coming years the majority of specialists will be female.

Most doctors practicing in the United States are graduates of US medical schools. There are two other groups of doctors in practice who make up a relatively small proportion of the total doctor population. They are: (1) foreign nationals who graduated from foreign schools; and (2) US nationals who graduated from foreign schools. (Canadian medical schools are not considered foreign).

Foreign Medical Graduates

Foreign medical schools vary greatly in quality. Even some of the oldest and finest European schools have become virtually "open door," with huge numbers of unscreened students making teaching and learning difficult. Others are excellent and provided the model for our system of medical education.

Tip

Any doctor with a license can practice in any specialty. Board certification is your assurance that the doctor has appropriate training for the specialty.

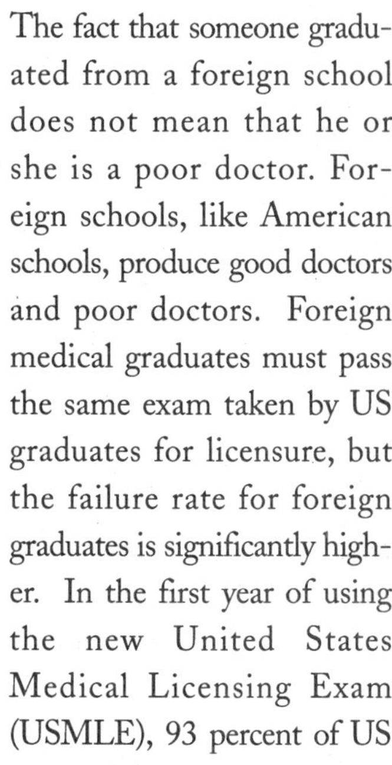

The fact that someone graduated from a foreign school does not mean that he or she is a poor doctor. Foreign schools, like American schools, produce good doctors and poor doctors. Foreign medical graduates must pass the same exam taken by US graduates for licensure, but the failure rate for foreign graduates is significantly higher. In the first year of using the new United States Medical Licensing Exam (USMLE), 93 percent of US medical school graduates passed Step II, the clinical exam, as compared with 39 percent of the foreign graduates. It is clear the quality of foreign schools, if not individual doctors, is not the same as US medical schools, at least measured by our standards. Nonetheless, many communities and patients have been well served by foreign medical graduates practicing in this country—often in areas where it has been difficult to attract graduates of American schools.

Residency

Most doctors practicing today have at least three years of postgraduate (following the MD or DO) training in an approved residency program. This is not only an important step in the process of becoming a competent doctor, but it is also a requirement for board (specialty) certification. Most people assume that a prospective doctor needs to complete a three-year residency program to obtain a medical license. This is not true in some states. New York State, for example, requires only one postgraduate year. However, since all approved residencies last at least three years and some, such as those in neurosurgery, general surgery, orthopedic surgery, and urology, may extend for five or more years, it is important to know the details of a doctor's training. *Simple* licensure is not enough of a basis on which to make a good choice.

The fact that someone graduated from a foreign school does not mean that he or she is a poor doctor. Foreign schools, like American schools, produce good doctors and poor doctors.

Without undertaking extensive and detailed research on every residency program, the best assessment you can make of a doctor's residency program is to see if it took place in a large medical center whose name you recognize. The more prestigious institutions tend to attract the best medical students, sometimes regardless of the quality of the individual residency program. If in doubt about a doctor's training, ask the doctor if the residency completed was in the specialty of the practice. If not, ask why.

It is also important to be certain that a doctor completed a residency that has been approved by the appropriate governing board of the specialty, such as the American Board of Surgery, the American Board of Radiology, or the American Osteopathic Board of Pediatrics. These board groups are listed in Appendixes C and E. If you are really concerned about a doctor's training, you should first call the hospital that offered the residency and ask if the residency was approved by the appropriate specialty group. If still in doubt, review the publication *Directory of Graduate Medical Education Programs*, often called the "green book," found in medical school or hospital libraries, which lists all approved residencies.

Board Certification

With an MD or DO degree and a license, an individual may practice any kind of medicine—with or without additional special training. For example, doctors with a license but no special training may call themselves radiologists or pediatricians. This is why board certification is such an important factor. Twenty-five specialties are recognized by the American Board of Medical Specialties (ABMS). Eighteen boards certify in 33 specialties under the aegis of the American Osteopathic Association (AOA). Doctors who have qualified for such specialization are called board-certified; they have completed an approved residency and passed the board's exam. (See Appendix C for an approved ABMS list; see Appendix E for the AOA list.) While many doctors who are not board certified do call themselves specialists, board certification is the best standard by which to measure competence and training.

You can be confident that doctors who are board-certified have at minimum the proper training in their specialty and have demonstrated their proficiency through supervision and testing. While there are many non-board-certified doctors who are highly competent, it is more difficult to assess the level of their training. Board certification alone does not guarantee competence, but it is a standard that reflects successful completion of an appropriate training program.

Board Eligibility

There are doctors without board certification who are highly competent, including many who have been more recently trained and are waiting to take the boards. They are sometimes described as board-eligible, a common term that is frowned upon by the ABMS. Board-eligible means that the doctor has completed an approved residency and is qualified to sit for the board exams, which may be given only infrequently. Most of the specialty boards permit unlimited attempts to pass the exam. Only the American Board of Internal Medicine (ABIM) continues to use and recognize the term board-eligible. The other boards neither use the term, nor sanction its use. The description board-eligible should not be viewed as a real qualification, especially if a doctor has been out of medical school long enough to have taken the certification exams. To the boards, a doctor is either board-certified or not. In some cases, doctors who have failed the exams twice continue to call themselves board-eligible. In osteopathic medicine, the board-eligible status is rec-

> ***Tip***
>
> *Rely on board certification to assure yourself of basic competence. Use membership in a specialty interest group to indicate strong interest and possible additional training in a particular aspect of medicine.*

ognized only for the first six years after completion of a residency.

In addition to the ABMS- and AOA-approved list of specialties and subspecialties, there are a wide variety of other doctors, and groups of doctors, who may call themselves specialists. There are, at present, at least 100 such groups. They range from doctors who are working to create a recognized body of knowledge and subspecialty training to less formal groups interested in a particular approach to the practice of medicine. These groups may or may not have standards for membership. There is no way of determining the true extent of their members' training, and they are not recognized by the ABMS or the AOA. While you should be cautious of doctors who claim they are specialists in these areas, many do have advanced training, and the groups at least offer a listing of people interested in a particular approach to medical care. Rely on board certification to assure yourself of basic competence, and use membership in one of these groups to indicate strong interest and possible additional training in a particular aspect of medicine. A list of these specialty interest groups may be found in Appendix F.

Tip

Ask a doctor if certification was awarded and when. If the date was seven to 10 years ago, ask if recertification has been granted.

Fellowships

The purpose of a fellowship is to provide advanced training in the clinical techniques and research of a particular subspecialty. In the US there are a variety of fellowship programs available to doctors, and they fall into two broad categories: approved and unapproved. Approved fellowships are those that are approved by the appropriate medical specialty board (e.g., the American Board of Radiology) and that lead to a subspecialty certificate. Fellowship programs that are not approved are often in the same areas of training as those that are, but they do not lead to a subspecialty certificate. Unfortunately, all too often, unapproved fellowships exist only to provide relatively inexpensive labor for the research and/or patient care activities of a clinical department in a medical school or hospital. In such cases, the learning that takes place is secondary and may be a good deal less than in an approved fellowship. On the other hand, any fellowship is better than none at all, and some unapproved fellowships have that status for a valid reason, which should not reflect negatively on the program. For example, the fellowship may have been recently created, with approval being sought. To check that a fellowship is an approved one, call the hospital where the training took place or the medical board for that specialty.

The subspecialty boards today tend to accept as candidates only those who have completed approved fellowship programs. However, since there are not enough approved programs in some of the newer subspecialties, such as critical care surgery, candidates are accepted from non-approved programs. This may be true in other specialties as well, and clinical experience is a heavily weighted factor in these admissions decisions.

Recertification

A relatively new focus of the specialty boards is the area of recertification. Until recently, board certification lasted for an unlimited time period. Now, almost all the boards have put time limits on the certification period. For example, in internal medicine, it is 10 years; in family practice, six, and under some circumstances, seven years; in anesthesiology there is no defined time period. In osteopathic medicine, all the boards need to set a recertification period by January, 1995. Many have done so already. These more stringent standards reflect an increasing emphasis, by both the medical boards and state agencies responsible for licensing doctors, on recertification.

Factors Contributing to Reputation

There are four important—and measurable—factors that contribute to a doctor's professional reputation:

- *Hospital appointment*
- *Medical school faculty appointment*
- *Medical society membership*
- *Experience*

Since the policies of the boards vary widely, it is good procedure to ask a doctor if certification was awarded and when. If the date was seven to 10 years ago, ask if they have been recertified. Unfortunately, many boards permit "grandfathering," whereby already certified doctors do not have to be recertified, and recertification demands apply only to newly certified doctors. Appendix C contains a list of the names and addresses of the boards and the certification period for each board specialty. Even if recertification is not required, it is good professional practice for doctors to undertake the process. It assures you, the patient, that they are attempting to stay current.

Many states have a continuing medical education requirement for doctors. These states typically require a minimum number of continuing medical education (CME) credits for a doctor to maintain a medical license. Twenty-eight states require 150 CME credits over a three-year period. Osteopathic doctors are required to take 150 hours of CME credits within three years to maintain certification.

> ***Tip***
>
> *It is usually best to be cared for by a doctor with admitting privileges at a hospital. Otherwise, if hospitalized, you will have to be cared for by another doctor.*

Professional Reputation

There are doctors who meet every professional standard on paper, but who are simply not good doctors. In all probability the medical community has ascertained that, and, while the individual may still practice medicine, his or her reputation will reflect that collective assessment. There are also doctors who are outstanding leaders in their fields because of research or professional activities, but who are not particularly strong or perhaps even active in patient care. It is important to distinguish that kind of professional reputation from a reputation as a competent, caring doctor in delivering patient care. In a consumer survey conducted by Towers Perrin, the management consulting firm, the chief criterion by which the respondents selected doctors was reputation. This was the most important factor for those enrolled in either managed care or indemnity plans.

Hospital Appointment

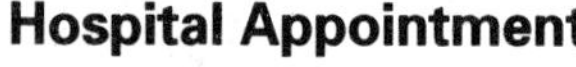

Tip

The best hospitals attract the best doctors.

Most doctors are on the medical staff of one or more hospitals and are known as attendings; some are not. If a doctor does not have admitting privileges or is not on the attending staff of a hospital, you may wish to consider choosing another doctor. It can be very difficult to ascertain whether the lack of hospital appointment is for a good reason or not. For example, it is understandable that some doctors who are raising families or heading toward retirement choose not to meet the demands (meetings, committees, etc.) of being an attending. However, if you need care in a hospital, the lack of such an appointment means that another doctor will have to oversee that care. In some specialties such as dermatology and psychiatry, doctors may conduct their entire practice in the office, and a hospital appointment is not as essential, or as good a criterion for assessment, as in other specialties.

While mistakes are made, most hospitals are quite careful about admissions to their medical staffs. The best hospitals are highly selective, so a degree of screening (or "credentialing") has been done for you. In other words, the best hospitals attract the best doctors. Since caring for a patient in the hospital is also often a team effort involving a number of specialists, the reputation of the hospital where the doctor admits patients carries special weight. Hospital medical staffs also review their colleagues to authorize them to perform specific procedures. In addition, they typically reappoint their medical staffs—and review them—every two or three years. In effect, this is an additional screening to protect patients. It is especially true of hospitals that have what are known as closed staffs, where it is impossible to obtain admitting privileges unless there is a vacancy that the administration and medical staff deem necessary to fill. Unfortunately, what a hospital appointment does not tell you is who on the medical staff is good, better, or best for you.

The reasons for a hospital's selectivity are easy to understand: no hospital, excellent or not, wishes to expose itself to liability, and every hospital wants to have the best reputation possible in order to attract patients. Obviously, the quality of the medical staff is immensely important in creating that reputation. Unfortunately, some hospitals are less diligent when a major group practice of doctors, all of whom have previously been affiliated with the institution, adds new members. In such cases, the hospital may almost automatically grant privileges without conducting the same intensive review given to individual doctors who are not members of a group practice. Also, some hospitals are less selec-

Tip

Doctors who are full-time academicians may be in the forefront of new techniques and research, but they are not necessarily better doctors.

tive in granting privileges when beds are empty than when beds are full.

A last and very important reason why a hospital appointment is an essential requirement in your choice of a doctor is that many states permit doctors to practice *without* malpractice insurance. If you are injured as a result of the doctor's poor care, you could be without recourse. However, few hospitals permit doctors to practice in them unless they carry malpractice insurance. This not only protects the hospital, but the patient as well.

Medical School Faculty Appointment

Many doctors have appointments on the faculties of medical schools. There is a range of categories from "straight"—meaning full-time appointment as professor, associate professor, assistant professor, or instructor—to clinical ranks that may reflect lesser degrees of involvement in teaching or research. If someone carries what is known as a straight academic rank (i.e., professor of surgery, without clinical in the title), this usually means that the individual is engaged full time in medical school research and/or teaching activities. The title professor of clinical surgery usually describes a doctor who has a full-time appointment in a medical school, but who puts a greater emphasis on clinical practice (patient care) than on research or teaching. The title clinical professor of surgery usually specifies a part-time or adjunct appointment and less direct involvement in medical school activities.

Doctors who are full-time academicians may be in the forefront of new techniques and research, but they are not necessarily better doctors. Nonetheless, you would be assured that they have the support of other faculty, residents, and medical students.

> ***Tip***
>
> *In most cases, an older doctor has more experience; on the other hand, a younger doctor has been more recently immersed in residency, the challenge of medical school, or even a fellowship, and may be the most up-to-date.*

When you are seeking a subspecialist, a doctor's relationship to a medical school becomes more meaningful since medical school faculties tend to be made up of subspecialists. You are less likely to find large numbers of general or primary care practitioners engaged full time on a medical school faculty. The newest approaches and techniques in medicine, for the most part, are explored and developed by medical school faculties in their laboratories and clinical practice settings. This is where they practice their subspecialties, as well as teach and perform research. Such leading specialists are not necessarily better doctors than community doctors—they are trained to provide a *different* kind of medical care. The best care is provided by a combination of primary care doctors and other specialists and subspecialists.

Medical Society Membership

Most medical society memberships sound very prestigious and some are; however, there are many societies that are not selective and which virtually any doctor can join. In addition, membership in many of the more prestigious societies is based on research and publication, or on leadership in the field, and may have little to do with direct patient care. While it is clearly an honor to be invited to join these groups, membership may be less than helpful in discerning whether a doctor can meet your needs.

Board-certified doctors are referred to as Diplomates of the Board. Some of the colleges of medical specialties (e.g., the American College of Radiology; the American College of Surgeons) have multiple levels of recognition. The first is basic membership and the second, more prestigious and difficult to obtain, is status as a Fellow. Fellowship status in the colleges is meaningful and is based on experience, professional achievement, and recognition by one's peers, including extensive experience in patient care. It should be viewed as a significant professional qualification.

Tip

If a doctor is board-certified, you may assume that assures at least a minimum amount of experience, but it could be as little as a year. So check the date of graduation from medical school or completion of residency if you want to know precisely how long a doctor has been in practice.

Experience

Experience is difficult to assess. Obviously, in most cases, an older doctor has more experience; on the other hand, a younger doctor has been more recently immersed in residency, the challenge of medical school, or even a fellowship, and may be the most up-to-date. If a doctor is board-certified, you may assume that assures at least a minimal amount of experience, but it could be as little as a year. So check the date of graduation from medical school or completion of residency if you want to know precisely how long a doctor has been in practice.

The one type of experience you should specifically want to know about is that dealing with any special procedure, particularly a surgical one, that has recently been developed and introduced into practice. For example, many doctors using a new surgical technique for removing gallbladders—laparoscopic cholecystectomy—experienced a high percentage of problems because they were not properly trained. This prompted new standards to be issued by the American College of Surgeons to make sure doctors using this new approach would be adequately trained. Do not hesitate to ask how frequently your doctor has performed a procedure and with what degree of success. Practice may not lead to perfection, but it improves skills and enhances the probability of success.

A consumer poll conducted for the Robert Wood Johnson Foundation identified office location as one of the two most important factors in the selection of a doctor.

Office and Practice Arrangements

Although clearly not as important as training or reputation, office and practice arrangements are usually of great significance to patients. Practice arrangements include office hours, office location, billing procedures, and office testing among the many factors that result in how well the office is run.

Many years ago, most doctors practiced independently in private offices. They were called solo practitioners and usually had agreements with other doctors to respond to their patients' calls when they were unavailable. In recent decades, most doctors have entered group practices; indeed, this is becoming the most common way for young doctors to begin to practice. Two or more doctors in the same specialty, or in different specialties (a multi-specialty group), share offices and staff to lower their costs of operations. They also cover for each other on rotation for weekends, evenings, and vacations. As a patient you may prefer one of the following: a solo practitioner who is covered occasionally; a group where you usually, but not always, see the same doctor; or a multi-specialty group where, if a consultation or referral is necessary, the specialist is at the same location. The choice is really one of personal preference.

Midlevel providers—licensed nurse practitioners and physician's assistants—have become more of a presence in health care delivery, especially in medical groups and HMOs.

There are other factors relating to practice arrangements that may or may not be important to an individual choosing a doctor. One is the location of the office. A consumer poll conducted for the Robert Wood Johnson Foundation identified office location as one of the two most important factors in the selection of a doctor. (The other was a recommendation by a relative or friend.) Actually, the site of the office can be very important in choosing a doctor you may visit on a regular basis. If the location is inconvenient, you may be discouraged from making needed visits.

Another important factor concerns the use of nurse practitioners and physician's assistants in the office.

Licensed nurse practitioners are advanced practice nurses in primary care. They have additional training beyond the basic requirements for nursing licensure, usually a master's degree or special certificate. They perform a broad range of nursing functions as well as functions that, historically, have been performed by doctors, including assessing and diagnosing, conducting physical examinations, ordering diagnostic tests, implementing treatment plans and monitoring patient status. Physician's assistants are licensed to provide medical care in many states. Unlike nurses, they may practice only under a doctor's direction and supervision. According to an article in the professional journal *Family Practice Management,* these "midlevel providers," as they are called, "can handle 80 to 90 percent of the problems that occasion office visits." These providers have become more of a presence in health care in recent years, especially in medical groups and HMOs. If you don't think you will be satisfied having your office visit and examination conducted by anyone but the doctor, you should determine up front how many midlevel providers are on staff and how extensive their responsibilities are.

Here are 10 additional questions that will guide you in assessing the practice patterns or arrangements of a doctor to see if they meet your needs. If there are other items not listed that are important to you, add them to the list before you make your initial appointment. You should try to obtain as much of the information as possible from the staff.

- Are you currently accepting new patients and, if so, is a referral required?
- On average, how long does a patient have to wait

for an appointment?

- Do you accept patient phone calls?
- Are you open on weekends? In the evening?
- Are lab work and X-rays performed in the office?
- Is full payment (or deductibles, co-payments) required at the time of the appointment?
- Do you accept Medicare? Medicaid? Worker's Compensation? No-fault insurance?
- Do you accept credit cards and, if so, which do you accept?
- Will you care for a patient in the home?
- Is your office handicapped-accessible?

If you have a chronic illness or disease, there may be certain additional aspects of a doctor's practice that could be particularly important to you. For guidance in such cases, you may wish to call one of the support or help lines, listed in Appendix L, if there is an appropriate one, to ask about what people with a problem similar to yours find important in a doctor. Some of these information lines can also give you information about doctors interested in a particular disease such as Parkinson's disease or lupus.

House calls also continue to be important to some people. Yes, some doctors still do make house calls! In fact, a recent *American Medical News* article suggested that 43 percent of internal medicine specialists and 65 percent of family practice specialists made one or more house calls a year. However, it is important to point out that house calls have declined not because doctors are lazy or arrogant, but because of technology, liability risks, and time pressures. Important diagnostic equipment often cannot be carried around in a doctor's little black bag and is only available in the office or hospital. Also, the time required to visit one patient at home markedly reduces the time available to see other patients.

The term "culturally competent physician" is a relatively new one describing doctors who have the skills and attitudes to deal comfortably with patients from minority cultures.

Personal or Bedside Manner

To many patients, once they have determined that a doctor is competent, the doctor's professional manner—also known as bedside manner—is the most important part of their choice. The Towers Perrin report cited earlier indicated that after reputation, communications skill was the most important factor sought in doctors. Patients want sensitive and caring doctors who listen carefully and demonstrate their concern.

What characteristics make up a doctor's personal manner? The four described below may, when considered together, give you a clear idea of whether a particular doctor will be your personal "best."

Listening

Professional manner includes the doctor's willingness to listen to patients, be supportive and understanding, explain procedures, and exhibit concern and respect. These skills are expressed at the bedside, in the office, or in any setting where there is doctor/patient contact. Listening is also a valuable diagnostic tool. Unfortun-

ately, these skills often have not been taught well in medical schools, and the lack of them forms the primary basis for complaints from patients. However, there is a growing emphasis on these vital interpersonal and communications skills in medical schools today, and with good reason. They are critically important to most patients.

Cultural Sensitivity

Some patients may prefer doctors who speak their language or are familiar with their cultural background. The term "culturally competent physician" is a relatively new one describing doctors who have the skills and attitudes to deal with minority cultures.

Ethical, Religious, and Philosophical Views

Religion, or at least views on issues such as abortion, utilization of life-sustaining measures, natural childbirth, breast-feeding, and other matters can also be important. It is perfectly appropriate to ask doctors questions about sensitive issues.

Decision-Making Procedures

Years ago patients took the words of the doctor as law, not to be questioned, or perhaps even discussed. That is not the case today. Consumers are better informed about health issues and may want to be actively involved in the decision-making affecting their health. Some patients do not feel this way and are comfortable accepting a doctor's diagnosis or course of treatment without question. Some doctors—in diminishing numbers, thankfully—feel uncomfortable with patients who want everything explained to them or want to be involved in decision-making. Consider how you feel about this issue and discuss it with your doctor to be certain you are on compatible wavelengths.

You and Your Doctor: A Team

Chapter 3

Trust and respect between doctors and patients have reached a low point in modern American society. A recent poll of consumers sponsored by the American Medical Association (AMA) concluded that approximately 70 percent of those who responded agreed with the statement that "people are beginning to lose faith in their doctors." (Despite concerns about doctors in general, much research has shown patients tend to rate their own doctors well.)

Trust between doctors and patients has declined for many reasons, including unrealistic expectations on the part of some patients and the patronizing attitudes of some doctors, which clash with the higher education level and medical sophistication of many patients. This has been further complicated by changing financial arrangements, particularly those involving the government and third-party payers, and the perception that some doctors seem to be motivated not by the values of the Hippocratic Oath (see Appendix B), but by those of the marketplace. The AMA poll cited earlier found that 69 percent of the respondents agreed that doctors "are too interested in making money." Perhaps a significant factor in creating this atmosphere is that the relationship between doctor and patient now has another dimension, the third-party payer. Another significant contributor is the huge amount of paperwork required from doctors. Generated by quality-assurance efforts, regulation, and complex billing, this burden reduces the time doctors are able to spend with patients.

Even while the doctor is responding to your questions, you should ask yourself:

- *Is the doctor paying attention to me and really considering my questions or do the impersonal, "stock" answers indicate that the doctor's thoughts are elsewhere?*
- *Does this doctor speak about good health and prevention with the personal knowledge of someone who seems to practice it?*

Given the formidable obstacles, it might seem impossible to find a primary care doctor who is well suited to your needs. If you have carefully read the preceding chapters, your work is half done. What remains is to find that special individual who fits the specifications.

The Initial Interview

When selecting a doctor, especially a primary care doctor, it is appropriate to request an exploratory interview. Frequently, doctors will engage in such brief interviews at no charge or at a lower-than-standard fee. Others prefer to handle them by telephone. It is preferable to find out about a doctor's credentials, office hours, and billing procedures from the staff beforehand so you don't waste time asking about basic facts. This leaves time to ask the doctor questions that will allow you to determine what kind of relationship could develop.

Ask the Right Questions

The most important aspect of this session is to see if you can develop a positive doctor/patient relationship.

Are you comfortable with the doctor's manner, style, and general personality? Do you feel a strong sense of trust in the doctor? Here are five questions to ask the doctor plus two questions to ask yourself that may lead you closer to a selection.

- What is your experience in treating _______(if you are seeking care for a particular illness or condition)?
- Are you open to treatments and therapies that do not rely heavily on medication?
- What preventive programs do you suggest for someone of my age, sex, and health status?
- How do you feel about involving patients in decision-making?
- What are your views on_______(ethical and moral issues of importance to you as a patient)?

Even when the doctor is responding to your questions, you should ask yourself:

- Is the doctor paying attention to me and really considering my questions or do the impersonal, "stock" answers indicate that the doctor's thoughts are elsewhere?
- Does this doctor speak about good health and prevention with the personal knowledge of someone who seems to practice it?

If your prospective doctor seems to measure up to your standards, get the relationship off to a good start by making an appointment for a complete check-up. During this appointment, you will have an opportunity to share your medical and family history and baseline tests will be performed to serve as a standard in the years ahead.

▼

One woman, imbued with her new "take charge" role in her health care, carried the interviewing process to the limit when she visited more than 20 doctors for exploratory interviews in the course of a single year. Each time there was some little problem: the doctor was behind schedule, the doctor was very brusque, the doctor discussed everything in complicated medical language, even one instance when she concluded that the doctor was just too young. Not only was she imposing on the professionalism of the doctors who conducted the interviews with her, but she was actually neglecting her health care; during that year, she never had a single medical examination. If a serious health problem had been in the developing stages, a year would have been too long to go without medical treatment.

▼

Tip

Always obtain copies of all medical records and tests for your files.

Talking with Your Doctor

After you have selected your doctor, your first appointment should include an extensive medical history. Your doctor should spend time with you, ask questions, and listen to your responses carefully.

Medical students are often told, "Listen to your patients. They'll tell you what's wrong with them." This conveys an important lesson not only for doctors, but for patients: *Good doctors listen, good patients talk.*

Analysis of doctor/patient conversations have revealed that most patients wait until the end of a conversation, even until they are saying goodbye, to tell their doctors what is really bothering them. This is just a small example of the dynamics of doctor/patient relationships. It is also a good example of a waste of valuable time—the doctor's and the patient's. One reason doctors need to be trained to be good listeners is that they frequently must ascertain what is troubling the patient not by what is said directly, but by what is said indirectly, not at all, or through body language and other signs. However, it is always easier, less time-consuming, and certainly more effective if a patient can describe problems completely and accurately.

Tip

Be open and honest with your doctor. Analysis of doctor/patient conversations have revealed that most patients wait until the end of a conversation, even until they are saying goodbye, to tell their doctors what is really bothering them.

Before you even see a doctor, you should prepare thoroughly. You should have a complete record of your medical history, including a record of X-rays and any other diagnostic tests, as well as blood workups. You need information about childhood diseases,

Patients want and expect doctors who listen, express concern, explain conditions and procedures in a clear and understandable manner, discuss medications and their effects and side effects thoroughly, return calls, are available when needed and, perhaps most important, spend sufficient time with them.

chronic conditions, hospitalizations, past and present medications, doses, and drug reactions, if any, and, if possible, something about the health history of your parents and even their siblings. Except for the last item, these are available to patients from their previous doctors or hospitals. That is why it is useful to obtain copies of all medical records and tests for your own files. Not only will this save you time and effort, but it may avoid additional testing and expense. Your doctor will also ask many seemingly personal questions about your work, education, sex life, and even drug and alcohol use. These are all part of a complete medical history and will help your doctor understand you better.

If you have a particular problem or concern, describe all your symptoms. Try not to minimize or exaggerate and, most of all, don't deny.

▼

An executive of a large computer software firm assured his doctor that he was "feeling fit," choosing not to mention the sometimes severe pain in his scrotum. Six months later the pain had worsened to the degree that it demanded attention. Unfortunately, the diagnosis was advanced testicular cancer.

▼

If you have questions to ask your doctor, make a list. Always bring a pad and pencil with you to medical appointments. When the doctor gives you directions, take notes or ask the doctor to write them down for you. If a prescription is written, ask about doses, side effects, efficacy, and alternative medications, as well as generic substitutes. The *Physician's Desk Reference,* commonly known as the *PDR,* is available in most libraries and is an excellent resource for learning more about medications. You can also get a great deal of information on medications from another health professional, your pharmacist. Do not hesitate to ask your pharmacist about side effects, generic substitutions, and other questions related to your medications. However, if the information you receive conflicts with that given by your doctor, consult with the doctor and follow his or her directions.

Research has shown the average wait in a doctor's office is 20 minutes. However, the doctor who spends extra time with another patient probably is the doctor you want for yourself.

A Matter of Time

Patients want and expect doctors who listen, express concern, explain conditions and procedures in a clear and understandable manner, discuss medications and their effects and side effects thoroughly, return calls, are available when needed and, perhaps most important, spend sufficient time with them. With increasing demands on their time, many doctors are left with an uneasy feeling of "running to stay in place." The end result may be a tendency, unintended for the most part, to rush through a patient visit. This situation contributes to the erosion of the doctor-patient relationship.

Also contributing to this problem is pervasive lateness on the part of doctors. Patients frequently complain that they spend hours in a doctor's waiting room, long past the appointed hour (research has shown the average wait is 20 minutes). Unfortunately, the duration of a patient visit is not always predictable. Unexpected delays may occur if the diagnosis is complicated or if a patient needs to discuss what is on his or her mind. The doctor who spends extra time with another patient is probably the doctor you want for yourself. If the lateness is excessive, persistent, and without apparent good reason, discuss it with your doctor and, if it is interfering with your relationship, consider changing doctors.

▼

After a delay of two hours in his doctor's office, one patient, a self-employed marketing consultant, made sure that it would never happen again. Did he have a showdown with the doctor? Did he decide never to return? Not at all. He simply made it a point to call the doctor's office two hours before his scheduled appointment to see how the schedule was running. Then he adjusted his own schedule to coincide with the doctor's.

▼

Strengthening Your Team

Chapter 4

When You Need a Specialist

For the most part, selecting a specialist is similar to choosing a primary care doctor. There is one major difference, however; typically you will be referred to a specialist by your primary care doctor. Suggesting a consultation does not show a weakness on the part of the doctor. On the contrary, the real weakness lies in a reluctance to suggest consultations when advisable. Your primary care doctor will receive a written report from any consultation or referral. You should get a copy as well.

Ask your doctor why this particular specialist is being recommended. Find out about the specialist's training and experience. If your doctor has sent many patients to the same doctor for the same treatment, you should find out how successful the treatment was and if the patients were satisfied. You might also ask if the specialist would be the one selected for your doctor's personal care. You should feel comfortable about seeing the specialist and, if you are not, you may want to find a different one on your own.

Tip

Your primary care doctor will receive a written report from any consultation or referral. You should get a copy as well.

Frequently, patients do seek out specialists on their own. If you are attempting to find a specialist or subspecialist without the guidance of your primary care doctor, use the various kinds of selection procedures described in Chapters 2 and 3. However, even greater emphasis should be placed on board certification in the relevant specialty. If you are trying to find someone to care for a very specific problem, make certain that the individual is well trained in that area. You may check to see if a doctor is board-certified by calling the American Board of Medical Specialties (see Appendix N).

You will also want to know if the specialist you select is well respected. The more complex and difficult the problem, the more important reputation is. In fact, you might well narrow your focus to doctors on the staffs of certain medical centers noted for excellence in specific areas. There are a number of books and magazine articles listed in the annotated bibliography that offer views on the best medical centers for specific problems. Last, make certain your doctor and the specialist communicate easily about your case. If you should have a problem with a specialist, or if you are not pleased with the care given, let your primary care doctor know about it right away.

▼

Easy access to specialists and subspecialists, especially in large metropolitan areas, presents certain problems in coordination that a patient should be aware of. This difficulty is probably epitomized by one woman who was treated by a dermatologist, an ophthalmologist, a rheumatologist, a psychiatrist, an allergist, a podiatrist, and a nutri-

tionist— all of whom had office space in her very large apartment complex in Chicago, thus eliminating her need to travel anywhere, or, in fact, even to put on her coat. Fortunately, all were quite competent and had all the necessary qualifications. Unfortunately, each was affiliated with a different medical center, which made coordinating her care with her primary care doctor very complex.

Doctors typically refer patients to doctors on the staffs of the same hospitals where they practice. There are good and poor reasons for this:

Why Doctors Usually Refer to Doctors in the Same Hospitals

Good

- *They know the doctors better.*
- *They continue to be involved in the case.*
- *Coordination of multiple specialists may be easier.*

Poor

- *It is easier.*
- *They will get referrals back.*
- *It reduces the chances of losing the patient.*
- *It may build social or professional relationships.*
- *The hospital may pressure doctors to refer internally.*

Second Opinions

Second opinions are a valuable medical tool, too infrequently used in many instances, overused in others. Clearly, you do not want to get another doctor's opinion on every ailment or problem, but there are definitely times you should seek out a second opinion:

- Before major surgery.
- When the diagnosis is serious or life-threatening.
- If a rare disease is diagnosed.
- If the diagnosis is uncertain.
- If you think the number of tests or procedures recommended is excessive.
- If the treatment suggested is risky or expensive.
- If you are uncomfortable with the prescribed diagnosis and treatment.
- If a course of treatment is not working.
- If you question your doctor's competence.
- If your insurance company requires it.

Most doctors will be supportive if you request a second opinion, and many will recommend it. In many cases, insurance companies will pay for second opinions, but check ahead of time to make sure your insurance plan does cover them. In an HMO, you may have to be more assertive because one way such organizations control costs is by limiting second opinions. This is especially true if you want an opinion outside the plan's network.

Often, the opinion of a second doctor will affirm the opinion of the first, but the reassurance may be worth the time and extra cost. On the other hand, if the second opinion differs from the first, you have two remaining alternatives: seek the opinion of a third doctor, or educate yourself as much as possible by talking with both doctors and reading up on the problem, and trusting your instincts about which diagnosis is correct.

If the diagnosis is the same but the recommended treatments differ, remember that doctors may have different solutions to the same problem—and both could work. For example, an orthopedic surgeon may recommend surgery to correct a knee injury while a physiatrist (a doctor certified in physical medicine and rehabilitation) may recommend rehabilitation. One might work better than the other or they could both work equally well. The choice may be based on your preference. However, remember surgical solutions can rarely be reversed. It usually is best to try a medical solution first.

Tip

You should always consider the possibility that alternative therapies may, simply because they are unproven, do more harm than good.

Alternative Medicine: Exploring Your Options

The *New England Journal of Medicine* recently reported that Americans spent some $13.7 billion on alternative treatments, estimating that 34 percent of all Americans used these therapies. The issue of alternative therapies is so important that the National Institutes of Health has created an Office of Alternative Medicine to examine many of these important questions.

One of the reasons conventional medical therapies are conventional is that most have been proven to be effective in a rigorous scientific manner. Most alternative therapies have not been tested under accepted scientific conditions—one, because they are relative newcomers in medicine and, two, because many of these alternative therapies don't fit into the exacting protocols set up in clinical testing.

You should always consider the possibility that these therapies, simply because they are unproven, may do more harm than good. The alternative approaches in use today range from legitimate searches and new therapies to outright quackery and fraud. Without the guidance of the scientific and medical community, it is sometimes impossible for doctors, let alone consumers, to tell the difference.

Nonetheless, doctors are becoming more open to the use of alternative approaches. One study reported that about 30 percent of the doctors questioned in the Los Angeles area said that they were open to alternative practices in one form or another. Medical schools are also indicating a new interest in studying approaches to health that may complement the strengths of Western medicine. Some of the therapies being explored include mind-body medicine, hypnotherapy, biofeedback, chiropractic, vital energy, metabolic therapy, naturopathy, homeopathy, therapeutic touch, acupuncture, prayer, and the use of herbs.

In the *New England Journal* study, 72 percent of the respondents who used unconventional therapies did not inform their medical doctor that they had done so. That is unfortunate, because such treatments could be greatly enhanced with the support and advice of a primary care doctor. More worrisome is the great danger that some people may seek alternative treatments in lieu of, rather than as a supplement to, more conventional and proven medical therapies. A classic and tragic example of this was the surge of patients who traveled to Mexico to seek a "magic bullet" cure for cancer promised by the drug Laetrile (made from apricot pits). There was no magic; indeed, patients lost money, hope, and, in some cases, the opportunity for timely use of proven treatment. If you do explore alternative therapies, be certain to let your doctor know about it. Some may be harmful, especially if you are undergoing another treatment under your doctor's direction.

How to Use Alternative Medicine Wisely and Well

- *Try to learn everything you can about the particular therapy you are interested in. Your local library may have material on alternative medicine. Many consumer magazines feature articles on alternative medicine, and the librarian should be able to direct you to these publications.*
- *Discuss your plans with your doctor. You might gain some insight into the therapy in terms of its possible risks. Furthermore, if you are currently under medical treatment, you should make certain that the two approaches will not conflict in some way.*
- *If you start an alternative therapy and it does not appear to be providing relief, or worse, seems to be worsening the condition, contact your doctor immediately.*

To learn more about alternative medicine contact the Office of Alternative Medicine (see Appendix L). To locate a source of reliable information on the practice you are considering, see Appendix L.

Clinical Trials: Should You Participate?

Each year, more than half a million Americans, some of them sick, but even more of them healthy, volunteer to take part in experimental trials of new drugs and therapies. Before drugs, vaccines, biological agents, and medical devices are made available for general use by doctors and their patients, they must go through extensive testing on animals and humans. The latter are called clinical trials. There is probably at least one in process at some medical center for almost any serious disease.

On the plus side, a clinical trial offers the opportunity for prompt use of a drug or other treatment that seems promising, and comes with the bonus of regular and thorough medical examinations at no cost to you (some trials even make allowances for participants' travel and other expenses). Moreover, patients are encouraged to discuss all of their experiences regarding the trial. In most cases, they learn more about their condition and, therefore, feel more in control, which can have a very positive effect. On the downside, you may be giving up standard treatment for something that may or may not be better. There is even the possibility that you will not get a drug at all, because most trials are conducted by the double-blind method, in which half of the participants get the drug and half get a placebo, or "dummy" medicine. Even the doctors conducting the trials do not know who is getting which.

What to Know Before You Get Involved

If you are considering participating in a clinical trial, you will want to know:

- Who is sponsoring the research? Look for a federal government, major health organization, drug company, or university-sponsored trial.
- Do any impartial authorities monitor the trial? Every hospital conducting research has an institutional review board (IRB) consisting of medical professionals and community leaders to approve that hospital's participation. There are also data and safety monitoring boards that oversee trials.
- Will there be pain or discomfort? Will diagnostic tests be involved? Both of these concerns should be answered in detail before you sign any form.
- How often will I be examined? The frequency of visits depends on the guidelines of the trial (called the protocol). Once your appointments are set up you should make every effort to keep them.
- Does my own doctor get a record of my participation in the trial? Routine health information is sent to your doctor throughout the course of the trial, but details relevant to a "blinded" trial are not disclosed until the very end when the trial is over.
- Is the drug in this trial approved for treatment of any other disorder? If the answer is yes, you then know that the drug has a prior safety record.

- If the drug is approved, will I continue to get it for free? Most drug companies will offer the test drug free to subjects for a fixed period.
- After the study has ended, if I have responded well to the drug, will I be able to continue using it, even before it is approved?
- Can I drop out?

If you are interested in participating in a clinical trial, make your desire known to your doctor, who can track down openings in trials conducted by drug companies, hospitals, private foundations, medical schools, or the federal government through the National Institutes of Health Division of Research Grants; the Physician's Data Query (PDQ); the National Cancer Institute; Current Clinical Studies and Patient Referral Procedure, NIH Clinical Center. A number of online databases also have information on clinical trials. An example is AIDSDRUGS, which lists substances being tested in AIDS-related clinical trials. A number of medical information services are listed in Appendix N and can provide the same information if you do not have access to or do not know how to use one of the databases.

Changing Your Doctor

Chapter 5

Obviously, at times there are good reasons for changing doctors. Some are very simple and straightforward, such as a doctor's retirement, illness, or death, your own relocation, or a change in your health plan. About 40 percent of people enrolling in managed care plans have to change their doctor to one who is affiliated with the plan.

An onset of a chronic condition may also prompt a change to a different medical specialist, such as a rheumatologist or cardiologist, if a condition does not appear to be managed well enough by a primary care doctor.

If you have continuing symptoms that your doctor has been unable to diagnose or if, after a diagnosis, your problems continue to linger without improvement, you should at least consider getting a second opinion and, depending on that opinion, possibly changing doctors. Doctors often have different approaches to the same problem. A different doctor may offer a different perspective and, perhaps, a solution.

You might also change doctors in order to find one who includes alternative medicine in the treatment or to find one who can help you enroll in a clinical trial.

People who have hostile feelings toward organized medicine tend to change doctors frequently; their complaints then become a self-fulfilling prophecy. They don't get continuous, quality care because it's impossible for anyone to deliver it. On the other hand, negative feelings may be prompted by unfortunate encounters with incompetent doctors or by the patronizing or otherwise inappropriate attitudes expressed by some doctors toward patients. Patients on the receiving end of such a relationship should continue their search for a doctor who better meets their needs.

Eight Reasons to Say Goodbye

Here are the eight most common complaints about "doctors I don't go to anymore."

Poor Bedside Manner

Good medical care is more than diagnosis and treatment; it's also an attitude on the part of the doctor that sparks a sense of trust in the patient. Being under the care of a doctor who is impersonal, abrupt, bored, arrogant, condescending, or sarcastic, may in the end be counterproductive.

The doctor's aloofness could have a more serious explanation: substance abuse or psychological impairment, which

Tip

If you have continuing symptoms that your doctor has been unable to diagnose or if, after a diagnosis, your problems continue to linger without improvement, you should at least consider getting a second opinion and, depending on that opinion, possibly changing doctors.

according to a recent American Medical Association report affects 30,000 to 40,000 physicians. Mood swings and detachment are signs to watch for.

Too Vague and Evasive

A doctor who dismisses problems with "it's nothing to worry about," or "let me take care of it," or who uses medical jargon isn't interested in having you as a partner in health care. The effect of this evasiveness can be anger, fear, and confusion, leading to failure to follow directions and failure of treatment.

Never on Schedule

Medical emergencies can make appointment scheduling an inexact science, but when snafus become chronic, it's a sign of trouble. An explanation can ease the frustration, but make-up time should not be at your expense.

Couldn't Diagnose the Problem

Some conditions can't be diagnosed on-the-spot. Others aren't attributable to one specific cause. That doesn't excuse an incomplete workup, however, which may leave you with a condition that could have been treated earlier.

Ordered too Many Tests

Sophisticated technology is available and doctors tend to use it, although some testing may not be necessary. The number of tests performed for diagnosis seems to be reduced in patient-doctor relationships where communication is strong.

Discouraged Second Opinions

A doctor who dissuades you from talking to another

doctor may perceive it as questioning his or her professional abilities.

Didn't Protect My Medical Privacy

No patient should have to discuss the reason for a visit, payment, or payment problems within earshot of other patients or staff.

Medical records can be requested by and turned over to insurance companies, lawyers, employers, and others without your consent, but you can certainly see them, too, to make sure they contain the proper information. In 23 states and the District of Columbia the law grants patients access to medical and hospital records; in other states, a doctor may let you see them anyway.

Unpleasant Office Staff

The staff takes its cues from the chief. A doctor who doesn't demand the highest level of performance from a staff may be sending a message about his or her own laxity in diagnosis and treatment.

Knowing how to end a relationship with a doctor is important. For one thing, you have to seriously consider what you will gain. Many patients are hesitant—and rightly so—to leave their doctors because they have no guarantees that they will find an improved situation.

If you're convinced that it is time to part company, you can do it gracefully (even though you are under no legal obligation to do so) with a letter in which you let the doctor know why you have decided to see another physician and request that your records be transferred.

You might even end up in a better relationship with your present doctor. Sometimes doctors aren't aware that they are in the midst of a deteriorating relationship until a patient wants to leave.

▼

In one case involving a woman in her mid-thirties, the doctor–patient relationship was severed over what was basically a conflict in personalities: the woman wished to have more control over her health care, and the doctor was reluctant to give it. The impasse was reached before the two could attempt any kind of a compromise, and the woman went off in search of a doctor who would better suit her personal needs. A year later, after a fruitless search for a doctor whose medical expertise she respected, she returned to her original doctor.

▼

Self Defense: Avoiding Questionable Doctors

In addition to finding good doctors, you also want to be able to identify and avoid doctors who have a history of professional problems. One way to do this is to make certain a doctor has not been disciplined by your state or, in fact, any state. You can call the appropriate state agency (listed in Appendix G) or check names in the book *10,289 Questionable Doctors*, published by the Public Citizens' Health Research Group (see Appendix P). This book lists the names of doctors who have been disciplined by states or by the federal government. The disciplinary actions were taken for a variety of reasons, including overprescribing or misprescribing medications, criminal convictions, alcohol or drug abuse, and patient sexual abuse.

Tip

The book 10,289 Questionable Doctors, *lists the names of doctors who have been disciplined by states or by the federal government.*

The Public Citizens' Health Research Group has been highly critical of state medical boards and their monitoring of the medical profession. The group's report compares state medical boards, ranks states by their disciplinary actions against doctors, and recommends actions for strengthening watchdog efforts.

The Public Citizens' Health Research Group believes that many states are not aggressive enough in monitoring doctors. They have been leading the call for public access to the National Practitioner Data Bank. The Data Bank was created in 1986 by an Act of Congress in order to track professionals who are disciplined for unprofessional behavior and to deter them from simply moving their practices from one state to another. The Data Bank became operational in 1990 and contains a record of adverse actions such as license removal, loss of clinical privileges, and professional society membership actions taken against doctors and other licensed health professionals, such as dentists. It contains the names of over 62,000 health practitioners who have either a licensing action or malpractice judgement or settlement against them.

There is strong pressure from some medical groups either to do away with the Data Bank or to place even stricter controls on access. They support their position with examples of errors in the handling of sensitive information. It is unlikely that Congress would permit the elimination of the Data Bank, however. In fact, it is possible that at some time in the future, access may be made more available to the public. You can write directly to the National Practitioner Data Bank (see Appendix N) if you wish more information.

A data service used by lawyers to check on a doctor's or hospital's malpractice history is LEXIS/NEXIS, the computerized legal information service. LEXIS will do a search and issue a report on any malpractice awards or settlements ordered by a court. The service is not inexpensive and the cost for a search can run to $65 (see Appendix N). Public access to the listing of malpractice payments is one issue on which doctors are very sensitive, and rightfully so. Many malpractice payments are made by insurance companies over the objections of doctors because the insurers feel it's cheaper to settle than to fight. Yet doctors who feel they are blameless contend that these settlements reflect negatively on them. Also, since so many specialists, such as those in obstetrics

Tip

People who believe they have a problem with a doctor, whether in regard to fees, treatment, or ethics, may contact the appropriate local medical society in the county in which the doctor practices, or the state medical society.

and gynecology, are subject to more frequent lawsuits because of the nature of their practice, doctors are concerned about how patients will interpret a malpractice settlement.

Tip

There is substantial empirical and anecdotal evidence demonstrating that confidence in the healer and the healing process plays a major role in many cures.

People who believe they have a problem with a doctor, whether in regard to fees, treatment, or ethics, may contact the appropriate local medical society in the county in which the doctor practices, or the state medical society. State health departments are also places consumers may turn to for assistance or information on disciplinary actions taken against doctors. The health department, typically, will only divulge that an action has been taken but will not give you any specific information about it.

Changing your doctor should not be considered a setback in your search for the best doctor to meet your needs. As you may have come to understand throughout this first section of the book, the personal and treatment styles doctors bring to their practices vary greatly. What is important for you, as a patient, to realize is that these subtle and immeasurable characteristics can be as important as clinical skills. There is, in fact, substantial empirical and anecdotal evidence demonstrating that confidence in the healer and the healing process plays a major role in many cures. Your main objective is to find the therapy – in combination with the professional who is providing the therapy – that works best for you.

Section Two

The Hospital of Choice: Before You Go to a Hospital, Know What You're Getting Into. Here's How.

Key Terms

▼ **Academic Health Center**

An entity comprising a medical school, one or more health sciences graduate schools, and one or more teaching hospitals. Academic medical center is a label applied to the major teaching hospital of this network.

▼ **Acute Care**

Medical care for patients afflicted by an illness that is sudden, severe, and not long-lasting. Acute care usually takes place in hospitals.

▼ **Chronic Care**

Continuing medical care for persons with chronic (long-lasting) diseases such as diabetes, arthritis, and lupus.

▼ **Interventional Cardiologist**

A cardiologist who performs invasive procedures such as implanting pacemakers. These specialists often have appointments in departments of both medicine and surgery.

▼ **Outpatient**

A person who receives medical care but is not confined to a hospital for an overnight stay or longer. Outpatient care takes place in hospitals, doctors' offices, and freestanding clinics.

▼ Palliative Care

Care for terminally ill patients aimed at alleviating discomfort rather than treating a disease.

▼ Tertiary Care

Highly specialized and sophisticated services, such as organ transplants, burn care, and neonatal intensive care.

An Inside Look at Hospitals

Chapter 6

American medical care is sometimes referred to as crisis-oriented medicine because it is centered around treating illness rather than preventing it. Doctors are primarily trained to diagnose and treat acute illnesses, with much less emphasis on prevention and long-term management of chronic disease. This means that most people go to a doctor only when they are sick rather than for regular checkups. And it often means that by the time many people turn to their doctors, their illnesses have become so severe that hospitalization is necessary. Thus, it is not surprising that hospitals have been, and still are, the center of our health care system.

The United States has the world's highest hospitalization rate—more than twice that of Great Britain and most other industrialized nations. Hospital costs now account for about 40 percent of total US medical expenditures. Since hospitalization was at one time the only way a patient could have insurance cover the cost of care, it was often sought by patients and encouraged by doctors. Because of this situation, America's crisis-oriented medicine has been largely organized around hospitals, but that has recently begun to change. Outpatient and home care are becoming more important, and managed care arrangements such as HMOs and other plans are placing greater emphasis on avoiding hospitalization.

Despite the emphasis on outpatient care, hospitals will continue to be one of the two dominant organizational forces in health care in the coming decades (the other being managed care) because they possess the resources—people, equipment, and facilities—to organize the delivery of health care, and they still monopolize the most sophisticated acute care.

One in seven patients suffers some problem directly attributable to the hospital. Among the problems are falls and other accidents, infections, adverse reactions to medications, surgical errors, and mistakes of hospital staff.

Hospitals can be lifesavers, but hospitalization is expensive and has risks, as well. One in seven patients suffers some problem directly attributable to the hospital. Among the problems are falls and other accidents, infections, adverse reactions to medications, surgical errors, and mistakes of hospital staff.

Obviously, no one goes to a hospital without a reason. Sometimes you have no choice, such as when you are involved in an accident or have an emergency.

When you do have time to make a decision, there are many factors to consider, such as size, ownership, sponsorship, accreditation, reputation, services, medical staff, nursing staff, equipment, facilities, cost, and, also important, location.

The following chapters will guide you through the process.

All Hospitals Are Not Alike

Chapter 7

Hospitals differ in missions, size, ownership, and sponsorship. Although in many respects they seem more alike than different to the average consumer, the differences are important because they often relate to the kind of care given.

Mission

The mission of a hospital is the most important characteristic in defining how it operates, what it does, and its "culture." First, all hospitals provide care. That is a basic mission. Most community hospitals focus on that mission, usually exclusively. Providing care is the primary mission of public hospitals, although some may also have a teaching mission.

Teaching hospitals, public or private, provide care and teach medical students and residents. Academic medical centers provide care, especially tertiary care, teach, and conduct research. While public hospitals carry the major burden of caring for the poor, all hospitals share that mission to some degree.

The issue of mission is an important one, primarily because people want to know if the quality of care in one kind of hospital is better than in another: For example, are community hospitals better than teaching hospitals? That is like asking which is better, an apple or an orange? The reason why the question is impossible to answer is because they are different hospitals doing different things. In other words, their missions are different.

A second reason making this question of which is better a difficult one, is that the names and labels are not always accurate reflections of mission. The following pages will help clarify all of this.

Academic medical centers provide care, especially tertiary care, teach, and conduct research. While public hospitals carry the major burden of caring for the poor, all hospitals share that mission to some degree.

Community hospitals tend to be smaller, and most have between 50 and 300 beds. Some community hospitals, however, may be larger, offering a full range of basic and advanced services and a choice of many different types of specialists and subspecialists. Most people receive their inpatient medical care at community hospitals. Typically, they are staffed with doctors in private practice who do not generally engage in teaching medical students or research. Most of these institutions are very well equipped, although they may not have the equipment and staff necessary to provide the most sophisticated treatment such as intensive-burn care, transplants, and open-heart procedures.

Academic medical centers and teaching hospitals are typically larger and always affiliated with a medical school, usually have 300 or more beds, and offer a far wider range of services. These hospitals perform the most sophisticated medical procedures, such as transplants, and engage in teaching and research. They are often called tertiary care centers because they provide these sophisticated programs.

They are staffed not only with primary care doctors and specialists, but with many kinds of subspecialists. For example, while the community hospital is likely to have general cardiologists on staff, the medical center may also have pediatric and interventional cardiologists. A community hospital may have general surgeons as well as surgical subspecialists available, but the medical center may also have surgeons who specialize in cardiac surgery, burn and reconstructive surgery, and transplants—all tertiary care services.

Some community hospitals may be larger, offering a full range of basic and advanced services and a choice of many different types of specialists and subspecialists. Most people receive their inpatient medical care at community hospitals.

Ownership/Sponsorship

Proprietary or for-profit hospitals are usually owned by corporations with a business orientation. Necessarily, their first responsibility is to their shareholders, and that obligation is to generate a profit. These hospitals may develop sophisticated protocols to assure greater employee efficiency and cost-effective use of expensive services, thus attempting to deliver quality care at a lower cost. Some critics are concerned that they may cut corners inappropriately at patient expense in order to reduce costs, or not offer services that are money-losers but which may be important. Others feel that by bringing profit-oriented management values to the hospital, they serve patients not only more efficiently, but better.

Voluntary or nonprofit hospitals are owned and operated by community groups, religious institutions (many of the nation's private hospitals were founded by Catholic, Protestant, and Jewish groups), or other volunteers. Members of the boards of directors are chosen by these groups. They are not paid for their services, and their role is to represent the interests of the community. The sole objective of these hospitals is to provide health care to the community, and since profit is not an issue, all resources are focused on that aim. Should there be any surplus, it is plowed back into the hospital's operations. Since these hospitals are nonprofit and thus receive exemption from many taxes, some critics have contended that not all nonprofit hospitals do enough community service, such as providing charitable or free care, to justify their tax exemptions. Some communities are now demanding that hospitals demonstrate their charitable nature.

In many cases, the public hospital is more than just a hospital located in a poor area. It is a primary care clinic because many poor neighborhoods have no doctors in private practice, and the hospital is the only source of care.

Public hospitals are owned and operated by governments, such as a city or county, or the federal government, which operates veterans' hospitals. New York City, for example, is a national leader in providing care for all its citizens, especially the poor, through a system of public hospitals. The Health and Hospitals Corporation, a quasi-public agency, manages a vast system of 11 hospitals, with 8,100 beds. Other well-known hospitals under public sponsorship include

Boston City, Jackson Memorial in Miami, and Cook County in Chicago.

Public hospitals often carry a large burden of caring for the poor, an important part of their mission. Because their budgets tend to be limited, public hospitals can be overwhelmed by their attempts to deliver this care. In many cases, the public hospital is more than just a hospital located in a poor area. It is a primary care clinic because many poor neighborhoods have no doctors in private practice, and the hospital is the only source of care.

Despite their challenging missions many public hospitals are known for excellent care, particularly in trauma.

The overwhelming demand can stretch the resources of public hospitals as well as their budgets, making it difficult to deliver quality care. Despite this challenging mission, many public hospitals are known for excellent care, particularly in trauma.

In general, many people within the medical establishment believe that nonprofit hospitals are likely to provide the highest level of care, although care may also be very good in many proprietary and public hospitals.

Teaching Hospitals: What Are They?

The label "teaching hospital" may be applied to true academic medical centers, to some public hospitals struggling to provide care, and to community hospitals that may have a few residents rotating through. True academic medical centers are likely to have more specialists available for consultation and are apt to offer the most sophisticated treatments and technologies. Not all teaching hospitals are academic medical centers. The best way to determine whether a hospital is really an academic medical center is by the nature of the teaching programs and the strength of the relationship with the medical school. The key to this is the number of residency programs. A true academic medical center will have a dozen or more different residencies. A major teaching hospital should have at least three residencies and preferably more. Hospitals with less than three residencies may lack the teaching infrastructure (e.g., full-time medical staff, number of residencies, and research programs) necessary for a "teaching culture" to have an impact on quality.

Tip

Not all teaching hospitals are academic medical centers. A true academic medical center will have a dozen or more different residencies. A major teaching hospital should have at least three residencies and preferably more.

Nonetheless, the differences between the services offered at community hospitals and medical centers are not clearly defined. Community hospitals are increasingly adding sophisticated programs, services, and equipment in order to keep up with medical centers. Health-planning agencies, state and federal officials, and business leaders have tried with little success to stem this competitive drive on the part of hospitals, which many believe adds substantially to health care costs.

Both types of hospitals can offer a high degree of sophistication and quality. In fact, many community hospitals have become much like medical centers in the specialization of medical care. With the tendency for doctors to specialize and subspecialize these days, and their availability in many larger communities, community hospitals have initiated services formerly found only in medical centers. This trend has been motivated, in part, by doctors who want to practice the specialized medicine they have spent time and money learning and, partly, it stems from the desire of many community hospitals to compete with medical centers.

Many community hospitals have become much like medical centers in the specialization of medical care. With the tendency for doctors to specialize and subspecialize these days, and their availability in many larger communities, community hospitals have initiated services formerly found only in medical centers.

Academic health centers are organizations that include a medical school and one or more teaching hospitals that provide treatment for the most severe and complicated cases. Many also include other schools involved in training health professionals, such as dental, nursing, or public health schools. The primary hospitals of academic health centers, called medical centers or university hospitals, are those a patient would be referred to for diagnosis and care of the most difficult problems.

It is not easy to determine a hospital's true mission by its name. Many hospitals today adopt the label medical center despite the fact that they are not really academic medical centers. Some say that such a term reflects their broadened mission, while others acknowledge it helps them in the highly competitive health care market. Both reasons may be true to varying degrees.

Tip

There may be a price to be paid for selecting a teaching hospital, which is that you should expect to be poked and probed by medical students and residents. If you are not comfortable with this, a non-teaching hospital is a better choice.

Different Hospitals: Different Care

The style of care often goes hand-in-hand with the size and mission of the hospital. In a smaller hospital, it is not unusual for a patient to receive what may be perceived as one-on-one care. Small, select hospitals, especially in affluent communities, attract highly skilled doctors, nurses, and other personnel who have the opportunity to focus on patient care.

On the other hand, because the larger teaching hospitals are dedicated to training new doctors, they have medical students and recently graduated residents involved in patient care under the supervision of highly skilled teachers. They also tend to offer the most sophisticated services, have the latest equipment, and attract the top subspecialists. There may be a price to be paid for selecting a teaching hospital, which is that you should expect to be poked and probed by medical students and residents. If you are not comfortable with this, a non-teaching hospital is a better choice. It is not fair to the faculty or to future doctors to refuse to participate in that part of the hospital's function, although some patients do.

One woman in her late forties, hospitalized for a six-week course of intravenous antibiotic treatment for endocarditis, an infection of a heart valve, was at first annoyed at the constant intrusions of medical students and residents at her bedside. Then she decided that she would consider herself a volunteer and that dedicating herself to medical science, at least for a limited time, might serve to improve the course of medicine in general. She found herself engaged in discussions with the young men and women, not only about her own condition, but about their aims and ambitions, hopes and dreams. She came away from the experience with a vastly improved impression of the medical profession. In fact, she is convinced that her positive attitude speeded up her own healing during the time she was hospitalized.

Another potential drawback of certain teaching hospitals is that some permit the existence of so-called "resident-run services." This means that the attending doctors allow the residents in training to provide most of the patient care without appropriate supervision. This is certainly not a desirable practice, but unfortunately, it does happen, and it is difficult to discover before you are admitted.

If you are a patient in a teaching hospital, be sensitive to signals that may alert you to this situation. Most obvious will be the absence of your own doctor. If your doctor stops in only briefly once a day, continually needs to be briefed by the resident, or does not seem to take the time to discuss your condition, the resident may be running the service. Although you may spend a considerable amount of time talking with residents, you should expect direct contact with your personal doctor as well as any other attending specialists.

If such contact is not forthcoming, it's time for a discussion with your doctor. Be assertive about having your questions answered. Although doctors are often overwhelmed by work, most of them want their patients to be satisfied with their care as well as to recover. If your doctor's response is unsatisfactory, take your complaint to the chief of service or the medical director. Of course, this kind of perfunctory care may occur with or without the presence of residents. If it does, speak up!

Specialty Hospitals

There are also hospitals that treat only specific illnesses or offer highly specialized services, including maternity, psychiatric, orthopedic, eye and ear, cancer, rehabilitation, or children's hospitals. They tend to attract specialists who are well-trained and committed to the specialty care offered, and they are frequently among the best for that care.

Hospital or Doctor?

There is a direct relationship between selecting a doctor and selecting a hospital. If a doctor practices at a given hospital, that is where you would be admitted. If you prefer a different hospital where your doctor does not have admitting privileges, you would have to change doctors. If you are in an area served primarily by one hospital, you will very likely select a doctor on that hospital's staff. In metropolitan areas there are usually many hospitals, and you typically have a choice. If you want to be cared for by a particular doctor who practices at only one hospital you will have to accept that hospital. If you feel very strongly about a particular hospital in your community, you should seek out a doctor on its staff.

If you want to be cared for by a particular doctor who practices at only one hospital you will have to accept that hospital. If you feel very strongly about a particular hospital in your community, you should seek out a doctor on its staff.

While our approach in this book has been to start by finding the best doctor, with the assumption that the selection of a hospital will follow, there are some exceptions. For one, certain problems may require the services of a specialized hospital, or one which is renowned for treatment of a particular condition, such as cardiovascular disease. In that case you may wish to investigate the hospital first. Another reason to begin with the selection of a hospital rather than a doctor is geographical location. If you feel it is essential to be in a particular hospital because of its location or the services it provides, you should contact the hospital to begin the process of finding a primary care doctor.

Accreditation: A Hospital's Objective Rank

Chapter 8

A fundamental characteristic of a hospital, and one of the easiest to learn about, is its accreditation status. While it is important to determine that the hospital is accredited, establishing the fact of accreditation generally does not reveal a great deal about differences between hospitals. More than 5,000 of the approximately 6,500 hospitals in the United States (about 80 percent) are accredited by the Joint Commission on Accreditation of Healthcare Organizations (JCAHO), which accredits all types of hospitals. Initially, the commission only accredited hospitals, but in 1987 JCAHO changed its scope and name to include other health care organizations. The accreditation of a hospital or other health care organization is based on a survey of the organization by a team of professionals including physicians, nurses, and health care administrators. Based upon the survey, an accreditation committee of the Board of Commissioners, comprising 14 members, acts on the accreditation decision. There are five possible accreditation decisions:

> ***Tip***
>
> *If a hospital is not accredited by JCAHO you should make certain it is accredited by the appropriate state agency.*

1. Accreditation with Commendation (covers about 80 percent of hospitals accredited. Deficiencies are

noted and the commission follows up to ensure correction).

2. Accreditation (with or without Type I recommendations).
3. Provisional Accreditation (generally used when an institution initially applies for accreditation).
4. Conditional Accreditation (recommendations and deficiencies noted are more serious).
5. Denied Accreditation.

Ninety percent of accreditation decisions fall within the first three categories. About 10 percent are referred to the accreditation committee for full review. That 10 percent includes all denials of accreditation and all determinations of conditional accreditation. Only about one percent of the decisions are denials, with the result that the Joint Commission has often been accused of being too lenient. On the other hand, denying a hospital accreditation could be tantamount to closing it and is not a decision to be taken lightly.

Tip

A fundamental characteristic of a hospital, and one of the easiest to learn about, is its accreditation status.

If a hospital is not accredited by JCAHO you should make certain it is accredited by the appropriate state agency. You can contact the state department of health to obtain a copy of the accreditation report. Some hospitals, especially smaller ones, may avoid the expense of JCAHO accreditation if the state they are located in has a comprehensive accreditation process.

Typically, a hospital will publish its accreditation status. You can ask the hospital or call the Joint Commission (see Appendix L).

JCAHO Goes Public

Although the accreditation status of a health care organization is public information, what is not public is the survey material prepared by the hospital and the Joint Commission report and recommendations. However, in November 1994, the Joint Commission began to provide the public with information on how well a hospital compares with other hospitals on 28 performance standards. The following is an example of how a hospital performance report is presented:

Areas Evaluated	Performance Area Score for GENERAL HOSPITAL Anywhere, U.S.A.	Percent of Other Hospitals Surveyed Which Received a Score Between:				
		90–100	80–89	70–79	60–69	59 or -
Patient Care Functions						
Assessment of Patients	73	77	16	7	0	0

Areas Evaluated	Performance Area Score for GENERAL HOSPITAL Anywhere, U.S.A.	Percent of Other Hospitals Surveyed Which Received a Score Between:				
		90–100	80–89	70–79	60–69	59 or -
Medication Use	65	73	19	7	1	0
Operative Procedures	86	74	18	5	2	1
Patient/Family Education	75	39	–	50	–	11
Patient Rights	75	21	–	13	–	66
Service Providers and Staff						
Medical Staff	64	26	11	25	16	22
Nursing	100	83	–	10	–	7
Staff Training	100	62	–	16	–	22
Physical Environment and Safety						
Infection Control	50	31	–	27	–	42
Safety	65	19	33	16	22	10

Areas Evaluated	Performance Area Score for GENERAL HOSPITAL Anywhere, U.S.A.	Percent of Other Hospitals Surveyed Which Received a Score Between:				
		90–100	80–89	70–79	60–69	59 or -
Organizational Leadership and Management						
Organizational Leadership	88	36	24	21	9	10
Governing Body	100	48	–	22	–	30
Management and Administration	100	35	–	17	–	48
Management of Information	64	69	24	4	2	1
Improving Organizational Performance	75	74	15	6	4	1
Department Specific Requirements						
Behavioral Rehab-ilitation Services	NA	74	–	16	–	10

Areas Evaluated	Performance Area Score for GENERAL HOSPITAL Anywhere, U.S.A.	Percent of Other Hospitals Surveyed Which Received a Score Between:				
		90–100	80–89	70–79	60–69	59 or -
Chemical Dependency	NA	38	22	10	9	21
Diagnostic Radiology Services	100	92	–	3	–	5
Dietary Services	100	74	–	24	–	2
Emergency Services	100	90	–	4	–	6
Laboratory Services	100	94	–	5	–	1
Nuclear Medicine Services	100	97	–	3	–	0
Pharmaceutical Services	100	97	–	3	–	0
Physical Rehab-ilitation Services	100	87	–	11	–	2
Radiation Oncology Services	100	100	–	0	–	0
Respiratory Care Services	100	88	–	6	–	6

Areas Evaluated	Performance Area Score for GENERAL HOSPITAL Anywhere, U.S.A.	Percent of Other Hospitals Surveyed Which Received a Score Between:				
		90–100	80–89	70–79	60–69	59 or -
Social Services	100	97	–	3	–	0
Special Care Services	50	54	–	16	–	30

This information will be available from the Joint Commission or from the individual hospitals, and you should seek it from any hospitals you may contemplate using.

Outcomes: A New Yardstick for Measuring Quality

The Joint Commission is also heading in an important new direction that places an emphasis on outcomes. Outcomes is a term used to describe the results of care or treatments. Unfortunately, outcomes studies have not been available to help consumers assess the quality of care provided by doctors, hospitals, and managed care organizations. However, that is changing.

In 1989, the federal Health Care Financing Administration (HCFA) released data on medical mortality (death) rates at each of the nation's hospitals. The controversy surrounding the release was great, and after three years the reports were discontinued because many hospitals felt that the analysis of the data was unfair to them since they dealt with sicker or poorer patients with higher mortality rates. *Consumers' Checkbook* magazine publishes *Consumers' Guide to Hospitals*, which is a report of this data from 1989, 1990, and 1991. (See Appendix P for information on how to obtain this report.)

New York State conducted an analysis of mortality during or immediately following coronary artery bypass surgery. The results were tracked in two areas, by doctor and by hospital, and publicly released for the years 1989, 1990, and 1991. This analysis is credited with improving the quality of care at some hospitals, despite the controversy it stirred. (See Appendix P for information on how to obtain the report on this study.)

While uncommon today, "report cards" that help consumers measure quality of care will be common by the year 2000.

There are additional efforts under way, led by business coalitions, HMOs, hospitals, health policy experts, and others to provide consumers with useful outcomes data—sometimes called "report cards"—to help judge the quality of care. Presently, the Joint Commission is working closely with providers, purchasers, and policymakers in developing an outcomes approach for measuring the quality of hospital care, known as IMS—Indicator Measurement System.

The Joint Commission is developing indicator measurements in eight areas:

- Obstetrics
- Anesthesia
- Trauma care
- Oncology care
- Cardiovascular disease
- Medication use
- Infection control
- Home infusion therapy

The IMS is expected to become part of the accreditation process as early as 1997.

Some hospitals, either under their own initiative or due to pressures from coalitions of large employers who want objective ways to measure what they are paying for, are moving to report cards. While uncommon today, report cards that help consumers measure the quality of care will be common by the year 2000.

How to Read a Hospital Report Card

As reported in *Business and Health* magazine, hospital report cards may provide consumers with outcomes information such as the following:

- **Patient discharge rates**
  Number of discharges in total and by specialty.
- **Prices**
  Highest and lowest average per discharge and per procedure.
- **Severity of illness**
  Per patient upon admittance.
- **Average length of stay**
  For patients under and over 65 years of age.
- **Morbidity**
  Clinical outcomes one week after admission.

- **Mortality**
  Actual versus expected number of deaths.

- **Inpatient care**
  Surgical infection rate; unplanned readmissions; unplanned returns to operating room; cesarean-section rate.

- **Outpatient care**
  Unplanned returns to emergency room; patient waiting time in emergency room of six hours or more; X-ray discrepancies; number of ambulatory procedures canceled.

- **Patient satisfaction**
  Percentage of patients who think overall service is very good, good, average, or poor.

Reputation: a Hospital's Subjective Rank

One certain measure of quality of a hospital is how many health professionals would choose to be admitted there for their own typical or atypical care needs. If you count any doctors or nurses among your social contacts, ask their opinions. You can also contact local rescue squad personnel or paramedics to determine how a particular hospital stands up in an emergency situation.

Health care professionals are sometimes privy to information that is not widely disseminated to the public as a general rule. Thus, it is likely that their subjective assessments are based on very objective quality considerations. Here are some factors that might make a difference to a member of the health field—and to you. Call the hospital's community relations department for information; unless the figures are poor, the hospital personnel should be happy to tell you everything you want to know.

- Percentage of board-certified physicians. Look for a minimum of 60 percent, preferably in the 70–80 percent range or higher.
- Percentage of nurses who are RNs. Sixty percent is a reasonable minimum, 75 percent or higher is preferable.
- Number of residents. The number of residents and residency programs shows the intensity of the teaching programs.
- Pathology lab certified by the College of American Pathologists.
- Mammography program certified by the American College of Radiology.
- Hospital mortality rate. This is a complex measure that is adjusted by patient risk factors. See *Consumers' Guide to Hospitals* (see Appendix P) to explore further.
- Nosocomial infection rate. The percentage of patients who get an infection while in the hospital. If you are considering a number of hospitals for major surgery, ask your doctor to obtain the rate for surgical infection at each one and discuss it.

Remember, even in excellent hospitals, the strengths of departments and services vary greatly. That is why it is important to seek out the reputation of a hospital for a particular specialty when you are trying to treat an especially complex medical problem.

Two Great Strengths: Services and Staff

Chapter 9

While reputation is important in selecting a hospital, it is not the only consideration. Reputations of nationally known hospitals usually reflect the reputations of their medical staffs in research and in pioneering new advances in patient care, and the reputation of their affiliated medical school. Such reputations may be accurate in terms of research and complex medical cases, but may not have any bearing on the quality of day-to-day patient care. Furthermore, not everyone can or would want to go to these nationally known institutions for most problems. They are expensive and may be farther from a patient's home than a good community hospital. On the other hand, for the most challenging problems, distance and cost are secondary to getting the best care possible. As the saying goes, a chain is only as strong as its weakest link; similarly, a hospital, which, after all, is only a structure, can only offer quality comparable to its doctors, nurses, and other medical and nonmedical staff.

Reputations of nationally known hospitals usually reflect the reputations of their medical staffs in research and in pioneering new advances in patient care, and the reputation of their affiliated medical school.

Services

The range of services offered by a hospital also is

important to consider. If you have children you should seek a hospital with a pediatric unit, and not all hospitals have them. If you have a serious heart condition you may choose a hospital with an advanced cardiology program or even open-heart-surgery capability. Choices such as these are typically made with your doctor. If you are new to an area and know that you have such a condition, you may want to select a doctor on the staff of a hospital known for a particular type of care. Usually, statistics on clinical activity are available from state health departments. Remember, as in the case of doctors, the more a hospital is engaged in an activity, the better it becomes at it.

Most acute-care hospitals offer a full range of services. They must compete to keep beds filled, so they need to maintain a broad scope of services and the latest technology in order to attract doctors and patients. While hospitals have been severely criticized for this competitive posture, they have had little choice. However, the overriding concerns about health costs and pressure from government regulators, health care advocates, and business leaders have forced hospitals to begin to explore greater cooperation in planning and introducing new services. The planners hope that greater coordination in planning will reduce the duplication of services and the expense that goes with it. Some cities have coordinated planning efforts that have worked. Typically they have been brought about by pressure exerted by a few major employers who are also major payers of health care bills. It remains to be seen if these models will be emulated nationally. Health care in most of the nation is still a highly competitive industry.

Ambulatory Surgery:
The New Operating Room

It is estimated that some 40 percent of all hospital surgery can be performed just as safely and much less expensively in a properly equipped outpatient surgery center. Procedures that have moved to outpatient settings include elective or nonemergency eye, ear, nose, and throat operations as well as certain gynecological, urological, orthopedic, and plastic surgery. The major benefits of these outpatient settings are convenience (by allowing patients to return home on the day of the treatment or surgery), cost-saving (by avoiding the expense of an overnight stay), and safety (by avoiding exposure to certain hospital infections). More than two-thirds of the nation's hospitals offer outpatient surgery today. Some 3.2 million procedures were performed on an outpatient basis in 1993. An additional plus: Since hospitals realize a substantial profit from these ambulatory centers, they are usually very attractive, if not elegant, and very well staffed with nurses and other support personnel.

Medical Staff

When reviewing a hospital's medical staff, begin by asking the percentage of attendings who are board-certified. The higher the percentage the better—at least 60 percent and preferably in the 70–80 percent range or higher. Then try to determine how much selectivity there is in the choice of the medical staff, since greater selectivity usually means higher quality.

Closed medical staffs are by definition more selective than open staffs. Ask if the heads of the clinical departments or services are employed by the hospital or are at least full time. Doctors who are full-time chiefs of service, or are at least given some compensation for that role, can spend a greater amount of time on quality and other medical issues. Ask to see a roster of the medical staff. If a large number are graduates of foreign medical schools, that is also indicative of less selectivity. Also, check to see if a majority of the staff are associated with a single managed care organization or other group. If they are, and you are not enrolled in that group, your doctor may have less access to the resources of the hospital.

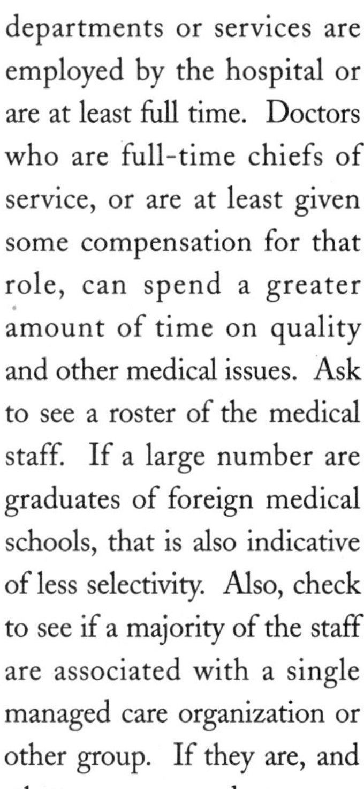

Tip

When reviewing a hospital's medical staff, begin by asking the percentage of attendings who are board-certified. The higher the percentage the better—at least 60 percent and preferably in the 70–80 percent range or higher.

Nursing Staff

Assessing the quality of the nursing staff is more difficult. One factor to consider is the ratio of registered nurses (RNs) to the total number of nurses (60 percent is a reasonable minimum; 75 percent or higher is preferable). All hospitals have nurses on the floor 24 hours a day, usually working eight-hour shifts. There is always one RN or a team in charge of a certain number of patients; in addition, patients may be cared for by Licensed Practical Nurses (LPNs), nurses' aides, and orderlies. Some hospitals have a reputation for good or poor nursing care. Such reputations are difficult to validate in statistical terms, but they can offer some guidance. The best way to check a reputation of any sort is to ask as many people as you can who have been patients in the hospital about nursing care and other aspects. On the other hand, you should always take such personal evaluations with a grain of salt.

▼

A recent patient in a large metropolitan hospital, a retired teacher, was pleased with the care offered by the nursing staff and didn't have a single complaint from day of admission to day of departure. This experience left her all the more puzzled about the judgment of a fellow teacher that the hospital had "the worst nurses in the country." As it turned out, the dissatisfied patient was really unhappy about her roommate in her semiprivate room, a woman whose large family visited frequently. When complaints to the floor nurse brought no response, the patient simply turned silent and harbored her frustration and anger. It would have been more effective if the patient had just reported her problem to the head nurse, the next up the chain of command. Better still, a polite request to the visiting family might have provided the quiet she desired.

▼

Other Health Professionals

These often behind-the-scenes individuals are a critical factor of any hospital. The support staff includes

Tip

One factor to consider is the ratio of registered nurses (RNs) to the total number of nurses (60 percent is a reasonable minimum; 75 percent or higher is preferable).

such important members as X-ray, blood, and surgical technicians, dietitians, radiotherapists, physical therapists, speech therapists, occupational therapists, recreational therapists, respiratory therapists, and many others.

Support personnel

These are the uniformed individuals who appear like clockwork to sweep, dust, polish, scrub, and leave a trail of that unmistakable antiseptic scent. Cleanliness is critical in a hospital—it keeps the infection rate low and, although they are not often given sufficient recognition, these people are important in the hospital's functioning.

Administration

Hospital, or health care, administration, is a demanding field calling for a variety of highly trained individuals. Managers oversee financial, housekeeping, and clinical services. Many have master's degrees, and even doctorates, in health care administration.

Medical director

A key position in hospital administration is the medical director or vice president for medical affairs (or similar title). This individual is an MD or DO who is responsible for the medical staff and, generally, the medical care. In any issue concerning medical care this is the top management person, who, as a doctor, has great authority and responsibility.

Patient advocate or ombudsman

An individual to whom patients can turn for help in solving problems with the hospital or its staff. Employed by the hospital, the person is also often called the patient representative. In some states, such personnel are required by law.

Other Considerations

Chapter 10

Even when you narrow down your choice of hospital to two or even one, there are additional factors that could sway your decision.

Location

If you have an especially complex and difficult problem, you may want to go to a hospital with special expertise in that problem, wherever it is located. Most major metropolitan areas have a number of major medical centers and specialty hospitals. However, for the most part, people receive care in hospitals near where they live. As a result, for most illnesses it makes sense to find a good hospital that meets your needs and is close to home or work, whether it is a community hospital or an academic medical center.

Equipment

Technologically advanced diagnostic equipment can improve care as well as increase costs. While much criticism is leveled at hospitals that own—and promote—such diagnostic tools, the reality is that consumers demand them and so the hospitals supply them. Some of the key pieces of major equipment you may wish to inquire about are CAT scanner (computerized axial tomography) and MRI (magnetic resonance imaging)—both imaging machines—in addition to the linear accelerator, used in cancer treatment.

Physical Facilities

The physical plant that houses the doctors, nurses, and equipment is important but is a lesser consideration than the hospital's services or equipment resources. You can get a sense of the facility by visiting to see if it is clean and well maintained. Unfortunately, serious physical problems are usually invisible to everyone but the experts. That is why the release of the Joint Commission recommendations discussed in Chapter 8 will be helpful.

As a rule, each state reviews hospitals within its borders and those reports are usually available under a state's freedom of information law. If it is publicly available, ask the hospital public information office for it. If need be, call the state agency for a copy (see Appendix G). These reports generally focus on facilities and safety.

Another, more subjective way of assessing facilities is to tour them. Again, ask the hospital's public information office for permission. They should provide a volunteer to help you look around. When you tour, observe the following:

- Is the building clean and in good repair?
- Is equipment stored properly and not unprotected in public areas such as corridors?
- Are traffic and access well controlled by security so unauthorized people are not wandering around?
- Are the staff members busy, and do they appear to be working with intent and organization?
- Is the staff courteous and helpful?

While an on-site tour may not yield a great deal of objective information, you will undoubtedly come away with the "feel" of the hospital, which can translate into comfort or discomfort as a patient.

Cost

Cost should be a significant factor in selecting a hospital but it is often difficult to get precise comparisons. One possible way to assess the costs of anticipated hospital and medical care is to ask a number of hospitals in an area their charges for a specific procedure, such as a hernia operation or an uncomplicated delivery, and compare the charges of the hospitals for the same procedure. Hospitals typically maintain a list of "published charges" or "established charges." These items are available to the public through the financial or billing office. Be prepared, however, for significant variation of charges by procedure or by diagnosis among hospitals, since there is no standard method for the development of these fees. Remember, the hospital charges for services or treatment include such items as room and board, medical supplies, and special services.

> ***Tip***
>
> *The best way to get cost information is through your doctor, who is, after all, your entry point into the hospital. Your question is simple: What will the cost be for this hospitalization and care?*

State health departments and the federal Health Care Financing Administration (HCFA) also require hospitals to file cost reports. These relate more to a hospital's cost structure than to what a hospital charges for its services. Although available to the public in most states, they are complex, lengthy, and difficult to use.

The best way to get cost information is through your doctor, who is, after all, your entry point into the hospital. Your question is simple: "What will the cost be for this hospitalization and care?" Since doctors are at the heart of the system, and have relationships with one or more hospitals, they can assist you in projecting costs. However, any estimate you receive is likely to vary—a little or a lot—from the final bill because it is difficult to precisely predict a patient's diagnosis upon admission to the hospital or predetermine the array of treatment, supplies, and services provided during the patient's hospital stay. Be sure to read Chapter 22 for a complete discussion of how to find errors in hospital and doctors' bills.

How to Examine a Hospital

Chapter 11

So far, we have described types of hospitals, how they are organized and operated, how they are accredited, and what major factors you should consider. In moving from the general to the specific, the following pages offer several types of checklists you may find helpful in selecting a hospital that best meets your needs.

Major Factors in Considering a Hospital

Accreditation

- *Importance:* A hospital should be accredited by the Joint Commission on Accreditation of Healthcare Organizations. See Chapter 8.

- *How to find out:* Ask the hospital public relations or public information office for the accreditation status. The information is also available from the JCAHO (see Appendix L). If not accredited by the JCAHO, make sure the hospital is accredited by the appropriate state agency.

Board-certified medical staff

- *Importance:* The quality of the medical staff is strongly related to the quality of the hospital and vice versa. Look for a medical staff with a high proportion (preferably 70-80 percent or higher) of board-certified specialists.

- *How to find out:* Ask the hospital public relations or public information office. Also available from state health departments in some states, as well as from the *Medicare Hospital Information Report* (published by HCFA) or from the JCAHO.

Salaried chiefs of medical service

- *Importance:* Hospital medical staffs are organized into various services, e.g., medicine, surgery, pediatrics, etc. These services may be called departments or sections, and each has a head, or chief, of service. If a chief or department head is paid to spend time overseeing the department, especially in larger hospitals, it usually means a greater degree of organization and attention to quality.

- *How to find out:* Ask the hospital public relations or public information office if the department heads or chiefs are full time or salaried, as compared with voluntary. Or call the office of the medical director or vice president for medical affairs.

Ratio of RNs to total nurses

- *Importance:* The RN is generally the highest level of licensure in nursing, although some nurses may branch out to become certified nurse midwives, nurse anesthetists, or practice nurses. A higher proportion of RNs to total nursing staff means the hospital is able to attract these professionals and is willing to make the financial investment in employing RNs rather than LPNs, a lower level of nursing certification. This factor has a major impact on the quality of nursing care. Seek a hospital with at least 60 percent of RNs or higher.

- *How to find out:* Ask the hospital for this figure or get it from the Medicare Hospital Information Report (see Appendix P).

Ambulatory care programs

- *Importance:* With a greater proportion of treatments and procedures moving to an ambulatory or outpatient setting, these programs should offer a full range of services, including surgery. Ambulatory care can avoid the expense and some of the risks of hospitalization. The key piece of information is how many of the various procedures are performed yearly. Again, practice improves quality.

- *How to find out:* Ask the hospital's public information office for a description of its ambulatory programs, especially for the surgical programs.

Location

- *Importance:* The importance of location varies. With a longer hospital stay, a location that is close and accessible can facilitate visits of family and friends. For a short stay or for a particular service, location may not be as important. Similarly, if you will need to visit the hospital on a regular basis, you should be certain that getting there is not such a burden that it discourages visits.

- *How to find out:* Test driving routes, parking, or public transportation when considering a hospital. Ask the hospital safety and/or security departments if any special arrangements are possible for regular visitors.

Costs

- *Importance:* Even if insurance of some kind is paying the bill, costs are important. A patient may be expected to pay some portion of the bill through co-payments or cost sharing.

- *How to find out:* All hospitals maintain a list of established charges. The list will describe charges for daily care, diagnostic tests, and various procedures, especially outpatient tests and procedures. Ask the hospital for a copy. There is also the possibility that the state health department or a local Blue Cross and Blue Shield Association or your insurance program has a list of charges.

Everything You Might Want—and Need—to Know About a Hospital

The following glossary constitutes a hospital's résumé. The definition of each feature includes, in some cases, why it is important to you.

Sponsorship

Denotes whether a hospital is public or private and who owns it. This factor may be relevant to concerns about religious principles.

Occupancy

Usually given as a percentage, indicates the portion of beds occupied, on average, during a year. A hospital with a low "census" (in the 30th percentile, for example) could have financial problems that might affect levels of care. A hospital operating in the high 90th percentile is close to capacity.

Admissions

The total number of patients admitted during a given year.

Discharges

The total number of patients discharged each year. Both admissions and discharges relate to how busy a hospital is; occupancy, however, is probably a more revealing figure.

Number of employees

Reported as full-time equivalents (FTE), this data is useful when calculated as a ratio of employees to beds. The number varies but tends to be between 3.5 and 5.0 for acute-care hospitals. Too low a number may mean too few staff members per patient and too high a ratio, except in a specialized hospital, may mean that the hospital is overstaffed.

Deliveries per year

Indicates the activity level of an obstetrical unit. As a rule, you can assume that the more people perform a task, including delivering babies, the better they are at the job. A figure above 1,000 births a year indicates a busy obstetrical unit. Below 500 is perhaps not busy enough. Of course, these numbers vary in rural areas.

Bassinets

Indicates the number of beds for newborns. This figure is related to the number of deliveries.

Neonatal intensive care unit

A special unit to care for premature or ill newborns. Usually found in larger hospitals, this feature becomes very important for pregnant women with a potential for difficult or high-risk deliveries.

Certified midwives on staff

Denotes whether midwives are given appropriate privileges at the hospital. This feature is important for women who prefer to have their babies delivered by a midwife rather than by a medical doctor.

Pediatric unit

The specialized unit for care of hospitalized children. Some hospitals also have a separate pediatric intensive-care unit. This is important for families of children with serious health problems.

Psychiatric beds

Indicates the specialized unit for care of patients who are hospitalized for treatment of mental health problems.

Burn unit

The specialized unit for care of patients who are hospitalized for serious burns. This type of unit is usually found only in a tertiary-care hospital.

Chemical addiction unit

Sometimes called a "detox" unit, it is a specialized unit for care and treatment of hospitalized chemically addicted patients.

Home care program

A specialized program dedicated to care of patients after discharge from a hospital. A hospital may directly sponsor or have a strong relationship with such a program.

Geriatric acute care unit

A special unit for the care of hospitalized, acutely ill geriatric patients.

Reproductive health service

A specialized program available to assist couples who are experiencing difficulties in achieving a healthy pregnancy.

Nursing home

An institution that provides continuous nursing and other services to patients who are not acutely ill but need nursing and personal services as patients.

Hospice care

Palliative care given to terminally ill patients, which is intended to alleviate discomfort rather than treat disease.

Hemodialysis

A process utilizing a dialysis machine to remove impurities from the blood in replacement or support of a malfunctioning or failed kidney.

Trauma center

A hospital emergency department specially equipped and staffed to deal with severe wounds or injuries.

Transplant programs

Hospitals may offer a range of the following transplantation services:

- *Heart:* Involves the transfer of a human heart from one individual to another.

- *Lung:* Involves the transfer of human lung tissue from one individual to another.
- *Kidney:* Involves the transfer of a kidney from one individual to another.
- *Bone marrow:* May involve the transfer of bone marrow tissue from one individual to another or, in the case of an autologous transplant, from an individual to him or herself.

Open-heart surgery

The correction of an inner heart defect or disease through an incision in the chest.

Cardiac catheterization

A procedure performed by a cardiologist, and involving the insertion of a catheter (a thin, flexible tube) into a vein or artery to recognize and/or locate blockage and to measure cardiac function. Catheterization may also be used to gather information about the circulatory system or to dispense nutrients or medication.

Physical therapy

The use of physical means such as exercise, massage, light, cold, heat, electricity, and mechanical devices in the prevention, diagnosis, and treatment of diseases, injuries, and other physical disabilities.

Equipment

- *MRI (Magnetic Resonance Imaging).* A noninvasive diagnostic machine that creates cross-sectional pictures of the body to provide images of hard and soft tissue as well as biochemical activity. This device is often used to detect tumors.

- *Lithotripter.* A nonsurgical device using shockwaves to fragment stones found in the kidney, urinary tract, and bladder, as well as gallstones.
- *Megavoltage Radiation Therapy.* The use of specialized equipment in the supervoltage and megavoltage ranges (over one million volts) for deep therapy treatment of cancer.
- *CAT Scanner (Computerized Axial Tomography).* A machine that carries out computed tomography, a type of imaging done by using X-rays and analyzing and displaying the absorption or transmission of the radiation by the tissues.
- *SPECT (Single Photon Emission Computerized Tomography).* A computer-enhanced X-ray technique in which patients are injected with a drug that emits a small amount of radiation. The chemical settles in tissues in direct proportion to the amount of blood flow in the area. Scanning, used in conjunction with a computer to produce images, is commonly used to detect abnormalities in the brain such as Alzheimer's disease and certain psychiatric disorders.

SECTION THREE

The HMO of Choice: When You Choose a Plan, You Should Plan with Care. Here's How.

KEY TERMS

▼ **CAPITATION**
A method of payment to physicians or other health care providers whereby a fixed amount of money is given for each patient served regardless of the number or nature of procedures performed.

▼ **CO-PAYMENT**
The amount paid by the patient for health care when the balance is paid by the insurer.

▼ **DEDUCTIBLE**
The amount incurred and paid by the patient before benefits become payable by the insurer.

▼ **FEDERALLY QUALIFIED**
HMOs that have been designated federally qualified have undergone evaluation by the Health Care Financing Administration (HCFA) and are deemed to have met certain standards of operative quality.

▼ **FEE-FOR-SERVICE**
Physician compensation based on services performed.

▼ **MORTALITY RATE**
The death rate in a defined population.

▼ **PREEXISTING CONDITION**
A physical or mental disability that a person had

before applying for insurance. Insurance companies may refuse to pay for treatment related to a preexisting condition.

▼ Preventive Care

Refers to health services that are aimed at maintaining good health and preventing illness. Such services include routine physical exams, immunizations, and certain diagnostic tests such as mammograms or Pap smears.

▼ Restricted Formularies

Refers to the drugs that are provided and approved by an HMO for prescriptive use by its physicians. The cost of drugs not included in the formulary usually will not be covered by an HMO.

Managed Care: A New Way to Take Our Medicine

Chapter 12

To the uninitiated, the term managed care might sound like a redundancy. For most patients, health care is managed, usually by a doctor, but sometimes by a nurse, therapist, or other member of the care team. But today, managed care means something quite different: In addition to your doctor there is very likely an organization, perhaps a profit-making business, that has a role in managing your care through the policies and procedures it sets.

Although it is a relatively new term to most people, the basic concept of managed care has been in existence since the creation of the first health maintenance organization (HMO). An HMO is only one type of managed care program. There are others. However, for the most part, we will use the terms HMO and managed care organization (MCO) interchangeably. When people think of managed care, it is usually the concept of the HMO they have in mind.

Nationally, about 19 percent of the US population is enrolled in some form of managed care. However, 64 percent of insured employees have some limits on their choice of doctors by virtue of some managed care element of their health insurance. Enrollment in the nation's 546 HMOs grew by 6.9 percent in 1993, according to Interstudy, the not-for-profit agency that tracks managed care. Approximately 47 million people in the US belong to HMOs, a fourfold increase from 10.2 million in 1982. The most rapid growth has been in the independent practice association (IPA) model, which now accounts for about 63 percent of all HMOs and 45 percent of all HMO enrollment. Insurance companies also now own more than one-third of all HMOs.

Nationally, about 19 percent of the US population is enrolled in some form of managed care. However, 64 percent of insured employees have some limits on their choice of doctors by virtue of some managed care element of their health insurance.

The growth of HMOs was stimulated by a federal law, known as the Health Maintenance Organization Act, passed in 1973 in response to rapidly rising health care costs. This act made HMOs part of the federal health policy. Basically, it allowed the federal government to mandate that employers with 25 or more employees had to offer federally qualified HMOs as a health insurance option unless they were self-insured. To be federally qualified under the law, an HMO must provide an extensive set of benefits and coverages. In fact, many of the concerns people have about HMOs are not reflective of federally qualified plans, which typically provide a higher standard of care and programs than do others.

HMOs are the best-known form of managed care, combining the insurance function and the provision of medical services. In other words, an HMO is a system for organizing, delivering, and financing health care. When an HMO accepts a fixed fee for providing all of a person's care, including hospitalization, it also accepts a risk. The HMO is projecting that the combined payment from all members will be greater than the total cost of providing the care needed by all members.

Because of this risk, the HMO must manage the care delivered to be certain the costs do not exceed the revenues. In most HMOs a patient selects from a panel of doctors or is assigned (although this is rare today), a primary care doctor. This doctor is frequently called a gatekeeper because of his or her role in controlling and directing patients' access to the resources of the HMO, especially to other specialists and subspecialists. It is this process, and the pre-set policies and procedures that govern it, which leads to the term managed care.

No matter how the health care system may be reformed in coming years, one of the most significant impacts will be on choice—of providers such as doctors and hospitals and, very likely, of insurance plans and coverages. Options are restricted in all forms of managed care; that is an essential element of this system. It is virtually impossible to control costs if users of the health care system have unlimited access to doctors and hospitals.

Although choice is controlled, it still exists. The trick is being able to choose wisely. For that, you need to be assertive and informed. You need to be educated about selecting a managed care plan, choosing doctors within that plan and, to the degree possible, selecting the best hospitals offered by the plan. As a well-informed, assertive patient, you have a far greater probability of getting the best care these systems will offer. The less well-informed, less assertive consumers, on the other hand, will get whatever the system delivers, good or bad.

Some Advantages/ Disadvantages of HMOs

- *A member's total health care costs are usually covered by one premium and may require only small co-payments—$5 to $10, for example—for an office visit.*
- *A patient is not required to fill out extensive forms in order to be reimbursed.*
- *HMOs are good for both preventive and acute care. A good program makes a concerted effort to promote the well-being of its members because it is in its financial interest to keep patients healthy.*
- *Some people believe that HMOs are weaker than traditional insurance (indemnity) plans in terms of chronic care.*
- *In all forms of HMOs, your choice of doctors and hospitals is limited, and you typically pay additional fees to use resources outside the network, if that is permitted at all.*
- *In many staff- or group-model HMOs, the gatekeeper is not a doctor but a nurse practitioner or physician's assistant. You may see them before seeing the doctor if, in fact, that is necessary. (Most of these professionals are well trained for their medical responsibilities, which are clearly more limited than a doctor's. Many develop superior skills, so their involvement does not necessarily mean you will receive inferior care.)*

Choosing a Managed Care Plan/HMO

Chapter 13

With the rapid growth of managed care, more and more Americans need to make choices among these plans and to make selections of doctors within the programs. This chapter will help you do that in an informed fashion.

When you are selecting among managed care plans, for the most part your choices will be from among HMOs of various types, so we will use that term most frequently. There are a number of important factors to consider; the following pages describe these factors, tell you where to find the information you need, how to assess that information, and how to use it to make the best choices.

The four basic characteristics you should consider when selecting an HMO are: model, coverages, cost, and quality. Each of these characteristics is summarized briefly, broken down into a number of sub-issues, and then explained in greater detail in the chapters that follow. The information to answer all questions posed should be available from the HMOs you are considering. Some of the information also may be obtained from accrediting bodies or from state agencies.

Model

One very important consideration is the model or type of HMO. Is it a model in which all of the doctors are in one central location (staff or group), or is it an independent practice association (IPA), with the doctors providing most care in their own private offices? In either case, is it a point of service (POS) plan, which allows you the option to seek care from doctors and hospitals outside of the HMO network? Consider which you prefer, and how comfortable you feel with each.

Coverages

HMOs offer different plans, and each differs greatly in coverages. Also, coverages are usually related to cost. If you pay more, you get more, but the relationship is not exact. In assessing different coverages, judge them as they relate to your needs and those of your family. A broad coverage you don't need is not of great value to you, but skimpy coverage for a service you may need often is a significant drawback.

Tip

The choice you make among HMOs should be based upon your *preferences and needs.*

Chapter 15 outlines the types of coverages offered by HMOs and describes what high-end (extensive) or low-end (less extensive) coverage might be for each benefit or service. These are just examples, and plans may offer somewhat different forms of coverages, but this chapter will offer you a guide for assessing each coverage.

Cost

Cost is related to coverage. In judging whether or not a plan is a good buy you must first assess the coverages as they relate to your needs. It is important to judge overall cost because while you and your employer may be sharing this expense, it is also important to judge *your* out-of-pocket expenses based on how you use health care. For example, if you're young and healthy and rarely see a doctor except for annual exams, a high-deductible or co-pay provision may not be a problem. On the other hand, if you have a chronic condition and need to visit a doctor regularly, a high co-pay for each visit may be a consideration. In the same vein, if you are on regular, expensive medications, the drug plan is far more important to you than if you are not. Consider carefully and honestly how you and your family use health care resources.

Quality

The issue of quality is a multidimensional one. We have divided it into three areas for consideration: accreditation, structure/operation, and outcomes. Each of these is examined separately. Quality is the most difficult characteristic to assess, but there are ways of doing it, and it's worth the time and effort.

Getting the Facts on HMOs

HMOs are usually very willing to provide prospective members with literature describing their mode of operation. When evaluating the literature, try to answer the questions on the following pages. If you cannot, call the organization's office. When you have answered all of them, sit down with your family and discuss the options.

The choice you make among HMOs or fee-for-service care should be based upon your preferences and needs. If you are not clear on these matters, call or visit the facility if there is a central location. A visit is a good idea in any case, so you can assess the physical plant, cleanliness of the facilities, and attitude and courtesy of the staff. In the case of an IPA model, visit the doctor you want as your primary care doctor. Ask questions and get assessments about the plan, including opinions and ideas from the people in the organization. HMOs, like other insurers, typically offer a variety of plans. Usually the offerings are determined by your employer, who in most cases is the major payer. Remember, most employers permit changes in health plans only during a selected period each year, often called the open enrollment period. January and September are popular, but not universal, times for these changes.

The material in the remaining sections focuses on a number of important characteristics you will want to assess when choosing an HMO. We previously raised the question of the model or form of managed care, and that is an issue you and your family should think through. The additional characteristics you should consider are related to coverages, cost, and quality. Finding a balance of all three characteristics is the key to your best choice of an HMO.

The Alphabet of Managed Care: HMOs, PPOs, POSs, and More

Chapter 14

There are a number of different forms, or models, that managed care plans adopt. It is important to remember that the various models have very different structures and doctor relationships and present very different faces to patients.

HMOs

Group Model

This HMO has a contract with a group of doctors to provide care for its members. The doctors' group cares only for HMO patients, and the practice is typically in one or a limited number of specific locations. The doctors are usually on salary. When there are a number of groups of doctors involved in providing care, it may be referred to as a network model.

Staff Model

The doctors in this HMO model are full-time salaried employees of the HMO and care only for HMO patients in one or a number of specific locations. Both group- and staff-model HMOs usually offer clinical, laboratory, and diagnostic imaging procedures at their locations and appear the same to most people. The major difference between the two is the employment status of the doctors. In the group, they are employed by the medical group. In the staff, they are employed by the HMO. To most consumers, the difference is insignificant.

IPA Model

In the independent practice association model, the HMO contracts with individual doctors or groups of doctors to provide care for HMO patients. The doctors practice in their own offices and usually see non-HMO patients as well. The doctors may be paid on a discounted fee-for-service basis (payment each time they see a patient or perform a procedure), or a capitation basis (a set fee to provide total care for a patient, including all visits and procedures).

POS Plan

The point-of-service plan is an option offered by many HMOs, whether IPA, staff, or group model. It permits the patient to opt for care provided by a doctor or hospital outside of the HMO network at higher out-of-pocket cost to the patient.

Other Managed Care Models

PPO

A preferred-provider organization may be a true HMO if it assumes the insurance function, or it may be simply a group of doctors and/or hospitals that have negotiated discounted rates, either capitated or fee-for-service, to care for a group of people. These doctors and hospitals care for other patients as well.

EPO

The exclusive-provider organization is similar to the PPO except that the EPO offers coverage only for the contracted persons.

PHO

The physician hospital organization is a new form in

managed care, and its name is descriptive. The PHO is an organization of a hospital and its physicians that can be a true HMO or a PPO. In many states, relationships of this nature between hospitals and physicians were not permitted, but that is changing. These organizations are still new, and their structure, performance, and success are still evolving.

Which Model Is for You?

In all of this alphabet soup, the primary questions you need to answer are the following:

- *Do you prefer going to one location for all your care? If the answer is yes, a group or staff model would be preferable. If the answer is no, an IPA model would be best.*
- *Do you like to see your doctor in his/her own office, rather than in a location that has many doctors and support staff? In that case, an IPA would suit you.*
- *Do you feel that you may need or want to go outside of the HMO network for doctors or hospitals? (If the answer is yes, you should consider a POS plan. If the answer is no, almost any plan would satisfy you, including a PPO).*
- *Is there one hospital where you receive all your care and where all the doctors you may need practice? If the answer is yes, a PHO may meet your needs.*

The fastest-growing form of managed care is the POS because it lets an enrollee choose care outside the network (at higher cost), and most people prefer that flexibility, even if they never use it.

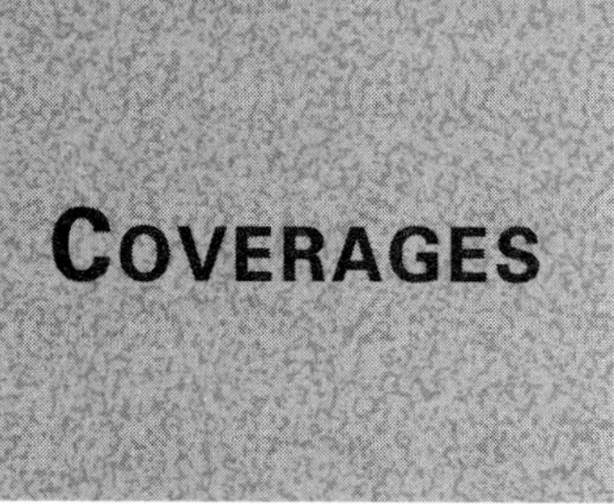

Coverages

Chapter 15

The following lists have been compiled to give you a sense of what constitutes minimal or substantial coverages. When comparing them with the coverages offered by a managed care organization, we suggest you rate each category on a scale of one to three. Since the needs of every individual and family differ, rate each coverage as it meets your needs and those of your family. Superior coverage that may not be important to you—for example, well-baby care for a single non-parent—should not be rated highly.

> ***Tip***
>
> *You should be assertive in utilizing your HMO's preventive care. You've paid for it!*

One important aspect of managed care is that preventive care is designed to be part of your coverage. When Paul Ellwood, MD, coined the term "health maintenance organization," the notion that costs could be controlled by reasonable preventive care was as integral an element of the concept as that of eliminating wasteful and unnecessary care. But preventive care is of no benefit if you do not use it, and many HMOs have not done well in providing preventive care to their members. A good HMO should be aggressive about seeing to it that its members utilize the preventive care offered. But if it fails in that responsibility, you should be assertive in utilizing it; you've paid for it! As a patient and a consumer, you need to be an active partner and assume responsibility for all aspects of your health care—prevention, cost, and quality.

One other important factor: We often assume that all managed care plans take care of every problem and to an unlimited extent. Not so! Be cautious—some treatments may not be covered by a managed care plan. Also, some plans may have a lifetime cap on the money spent for an individual's care—such as a million-dollar cap. Check on this, just as you would for an indemnity plan.

▼

The owner of a small service business set out to provide health coverage for his small staff of three. He examined the sales packages from several managed care organizations and finally decided to enroll his firm with an HMO that listed both a primary care doctor and an orthopedic specialist who were familiar to him. Some time after joining the HMO, the businessman injured his knee and saw the primary care doctor for an initial examination. When it became obvious that orthopedic care would be necessary, he was surprised to learn that the orthopedist accepted referrals only from particular primary care doctors in the HMO, leaving the patient to seek care from a different orthopedist whose credentials were not known to him and at a hospital that was unfamiliar.

▼

After you have examined all of the coverages, compare competing plans on the basis of coverages, cost, and quality to select the best one for you and your family.

The following list describes a range of coverages offered by managed care plans. Each is accompanied by two examples. One example may be considered a "high-end" benefit and the other a "low-end" benefit. These examples can provide you with a point of reference to judge the quality of benefits offered by plans you are considering. However, remember that price is a consideration when comparing coverages, and the HMOs you are considering may structure their coverages differently than these examples.

Coverage

Key

▲ High-End Plan

▼ Low-End Plan

Physical exams

▲ 100% coverage for routine checkups

▼ Coverage for exams due to illness or injury

Note: Some HMOs allow annual exams for members through age 19 and over 51, and include women's gynecological exams and Pap smears. Otherwise, exams are restricted to every five years for those 20–40 years old and every two years for those 41-50.

Preexisting conditions

▲ Delay in coverage of 12 to 24 months after contract effective date

▼ Denial of coverage

Dependent definition

▲▼

Usually includes spouse under age 65 and unmarried children up to age 19 or 24 if considered dependents for federal income tax purposes

Eye and ear exams

▲ Routine coverage

▼ Coverage for those under 18 years or due to illness or injury

Note: Co-pay usually applies.

Prenatal and postnatal care

▲ 100% coverage

▼ 100% coverage after $1,000 co-pay for professional services, 80% coverage for hospital services

Family planning (tubal ligation, vasectomies, contraceptives and natural methods)

▲▼

Varies

Elective abortion

▲ Co-pay ranging from $100

▼ No coverage

Well-baby care

▲▼

From birth through age two most HMOs provide 100% coverage (some with co-pay) for checkups. Ages three-19, most HMOs provide 100% coverage (some with co-pay) of annual checkups

Allergy tests and treatment

▲ Complete coverage

▼ $50 co-pay for testing

Wellness programs

▲▼

Usually authorized and provided at no cost to members by the HMO. Can include a range of health education and health promotion services such as newsletters, resource guides, classes, and courses. Some HMOs provide their members with discounted rates at health clubs.

Physical therapy

▲ 60 visits per year

▼ 20 visits per year

Note: Co-pay often applies.

Mental health—inpatient

▲ Unlimited coverage in hospital and 60 days per year in psychiatric hospital

▼ 30 days annually or 190 days lifetime

Mental health—outpatient

▲ Unlimited coverage

▼ 20 individual visits annually, 40 group visits

Note: Co-pay often applies.

Substance abuse program—inpatient

▲ Unlimited coverage

▼ 20 days coverage per year

Note: Co-pay often applies.

Substance abuse program—outpatient

▲ Unlimited coverage
▼ 30 days coverage per year

Surgery

▲ 100% coverage
▼ 75% coverage

Outside second opinion

▲ 40% coverage
▼ No coverage

Note: Only as authorized.

Diagnostic tests – outpatient (laboratory, X-rays, MRIs, CAT scans)

▲ 100% coverage
▼ Co-pay requirement

Home health care

▲ 180 visits per year
▼ 20 visits per year

Note: Co-pay often applies; restrictions as to providers.

Extended care coverage

▲ 120 days per year
▼ 30 days per year

Note: Some HMOs may put a cap on total amount spent annually; co-pay often applies, from $20 to $50 per day.

Emergency/urgent care

▲ 100% coverage
▼ 75% coverage

Note: Co-pay ranging from $50 to $100 can apply; an HMO may require prior notification before care is sought, and care may have to be received at an affiliated facility.

Organ transplants

▲ Usually includes corneal, bone marrow, kidney, and liver. In some cases, heart, lung, kidney, and pancreas are included.

Note: Special permission may be required; co-pay applies.

Ambulance services

▲ 100% coverage

▼ 75% coverage

Occupational therapy

▲ 60 days coverage per year

▼ 20 days coverage per year

Note: Co-pay often applies.

Speech therapy

▲ 60 days coverage per year

▼ 20 days coverage per year

Note: Co-pay often applies.

Prosthetics

▲ 80% coverage

▼ 50% coverage

Medical equipment

▲ 80% coverage
▼ 50% coverage

Podiatry

▲ Complete coverage with co-pay
▼ Limited (cutting procedures only)

Chiropractic

▲ Complete coverage with co-pay
▼ Limited (new injuries only)

Dental care

▲ Complete coverage for children under 12
▼ Preventive care only

Note: Complete coverage for other than children is usually only available with a rider.

Prescription drugs

▲ 90–day mail order supply
▼ 30–day supply

Note: Co-pay ranges from $2 to $10 per prescription; HMOs often require prescriptions to be filled from their own formularies (list of drugs).

Consultations

▲ 100% coverage
▼ Co-pay

Note: Usually covered as any other office visit.

Area of service

▲▼
Usually regional; some national networks offer care outside immediate area on a temporary basis

Out-of-network

▲▼
Usually only for emergency or urgent care coverage

Note: Some HMOs will pay a portion of non-urgent out-of-network care up to 40%.

Maximum lifetime

▲ Unlimited benefit
▼ $1 million lifetime benefit

Costs: How You Pay for Managed Care

Chapter 16

The fixed fee paid to an HMO for coverage is generally called a premium. In 1994, according to a study by Applied Benefits Research, Inc., the average monthly charge for an individual was $153.94 and for a family, $441.79.

The rate of increase in managed care charges in recent years has been lower than increases for other health insurance. HMO premiums, for instance, rose an average of 5 percent for families in 1993, while the average rate of increase for other health insurance plans was 6 percent. However, POS plans had a rate increase of only 4.9 percent.

HMOs generally are able to keep down costs through fewer hospitalizations and shorter stays for those who are hospitalized. Outpatient surgery is preferred whenever it is medically feasible. Studies have shown that HMO members are hospitalized roughly half as often as comparable groups. Managed care programs also control their *own* costs better. *Fortune* reported that operating costs of HMOs are increasing no more than 3 percent annually vs. 7 percent to 12 percent for the operations of traditional insurance companies.

The premium generally covers almost all your care. There are very limited or no deductibles and no co-insurance. Many plans do, however, have a slight charge or co-payment for each office visit and for prescription drugs.

Most important, don't assume that all HMOs take care of every medical problem and to an unlimited extent. Some treatments may not be covered by an HMO. Also, some plans may have a lifetime cap on the money spent for an individual's care, such as a million-dollar cap. Be alert as you consider your choices in any type of managed care plan. Check on the extent of your coverage, just as you would for an indemnity plan.

Tip

For hospitalization, HMOs generally cover all expenses, while many private health insurance plans have ceilings on dollar payments and limits on the maximum number of days of hospitalization.

The monthly premium paid to an HMO could be higher than the premium charged by a private commercial insurance carrier. However, to make a true cost comparison between the two kinds of coverage, you have to look at more than the premium.

A commercial health insurance plan, for instance, may include a $100 to $1,000 or higher annual deductible. Each year you must pay medical bills up to the level of the deductible before the insurance plan reimburses you for further medical expenses.

In addition, most major medical insurance covers 80 percent of eligible services; you pay the other 20 percent, generally up to a cap. Also, routine physical examinations, and often other preventive care, are not usually covered by private insurance. For hospitalization, HMOs generally cover all expenses, while many private health insurance plans have ceilings on dollar payments and limits on the maximum number of days of hospitalization.

Whether an HMO in the long run costs you and your family less than a traditional insurance plan depends on how much you use medical services. In most cases, however, you should save money since there are so few out-of-pocket expenses. The premium—often paid totally or partially by your employer—should cover most of your treatment.

If you belong to a federally qualified plan and your employer pays all or a part of the premium, the employer contribution must be at least equal to the amount contributed to the main health insurance plan offered by the company. If you pay a share of the cost, your employer must give you the opportunity to have your share deducted from your paycheck.

Payment: Important Points to Consider

- How much is deducted from your paycheck each month for health insurance?
- How much do you pay for an office visit to the doctor? For prescriptions?
- If you are treated by a doctor not participating in the plan, how much do you pay?
- What are the procedures and time frame for reimbursement for any out-of-pocket expenses?
- If non-network doctors bill for service, do they bill you directly or do they bill the plan?

- What is the total amount you must pay before you reach your deductible limit?
- How high is the lifetime maximum and is it high enough? (A million dollars should be considered a minimum.)
- What is the fixed fee for individuals and for families? When was the last premium increase? How do recent increases compare with other managed care plans and other insurance plans offered by your employer?
- What will your employer's contribution be and is that contribution the same for all health plans offered?
- If you must use a non-plan hospital in an emergency, how quickly must you file a claim and how long on average will you have to wait for reimbursement?

In our review of over 50 different managed care plans, primarily HMOs, it was clear that the price of each differed dramatically and was usually related to the coverages offered. The table on the following page shows examples of expensive and less expensive plans. But prices cannot be judged in isolation. When you are examining the cost question, do so in the manner described on these pages.

Can Managed Care Control Costs?

Advocates can find studies to support either the proposition that managed care controls costs or that it does not. However, on the whole, the preponderance of reports suggest that managed care can and does control costs.

HMO Cost Comparisons: a Reference Guide

	High	Low
Family monthly premium	$918	$296
Individual monthly premium	$516	$105
Co-payment	$15	$5
Drug co-pay, per prescription	$10	$2
Yearly co-pay maximum	$3,000	$0

Those who maintain that managed care does not produce an overall reduction in health care costs attribute the illusory lower cost of managed care to "skimming" or "cherry picking," a practice whereby a provider enrolls or selects younger, healthier members who use fewer health care resources. The converse of this skimming is known as adverse selection, in which the older, less healthy population ends up in the same insurance pools. It has been shown that people under the age of 45, who generally use fewer health care resources, do show a greater preference for HMOs.

Some studies suggest that costs may be reduced at first, but they eventually begin to rise again after initial cost savings have been taken. Other studies have shown different results, but even if you take only 10 percent to 15 percent out of a family's or a business's health care bill, that is a significant savings. According to a survey conducted by the benefits consulting firm, Towers Perrin, premiums for HMO plans rose by 5 percent from 1993 to 1994, while premiums for indemnity plans rose by 6 percent in the same period. Some HMO plans may be more expensive than indemnity plans, but that is usually due to more complete coverages and lower-cost office visits in the form of co-pays.

Those who feel that managed care organizations do not control costs are a diminishing number. The debate on the cost side of managed care is lessening, but the debate about quality continues.

Grading Managed Care: Quality

Chapter 17

As with any insurance plan, when selecting an HMO you want to consider cost, quality, and coverages. The factor of quality is especially important in managed care because the plan doesn't just dictate to what extent medical procedures are paid for; it is actually providing health care. While the goal of this chapter is to provide you with an outline for comparing one HMO with another, the question of quality is also raised when people discuss HMOs as compared with traditional indemnity insurance. Despite the concerns voiced by some critics, there is no evidence that enrollees in HMOs, or other kinds of managed care plans, receive poorer health care than people covered by traditional indemnity insurance. In fact, the supporters of HMOs believe that managed care can improve quality through an emphasis on prevention. There are three dimensions of quality we will explore in the following chapters: accreditation, structure and operation, and outcomes. These will be explained so that you can use them, alone or in combination, to help you select the highest-quality managed care program for you and your family.

Tip

Supporters of HMOs believe that managed care can improve quality through an emphasis on prevention.

Accreditation

Like hospitals, HMOs and other managed care organizations may be accredited.

Two organizations are involved in accrediting managed care organizations: the National Committee for Quality Assurance (NCQA) and the Joint Commission on Accreditation of Healthcare Organizations (JCAHO).

The National Committee for Quality Assurance has developed standards for accrediting managed care organizations that focus on six areas: quality improvement, utilization management, credentiality, members' rights and responsibilities, preventive care service guidelines, and medical records.

Managed care organizations may apply for accreditation by asking for a survey based on the criteria outlined in the Standards of Accreditations. Experienced managed care professionals, including doctors, make up the survey team. Accreditation is awarded for a three-year period, unless revoked, after which a new survey and accreditation review is undertaken. Under the NCQA, there are five possible decisions:

1. Full accreditation
2. Accreditation with commendation
3. Provisional accreditation
4. Denial/revocation of accredited status
5. Deferral of accreditation

Thus far, only 133 of the nation's 546 HMOs have been accredited, while 156 have been reviewed. NCQA also accredits many forms of managed care including POS plans, group HMOs, staff HMOs, IPAs, and mixed models. Since relatively few managed care organizations are accredited, it is clear that accreditation is still a new and not widely accepted concept, but that is changing. Nonetheless, 19 million people, or 42 percent of the population enrolled in managed care, are members of the 156 managed care plans that have been reviewed. With the urging of the Robert Wood Johnson Foundation, which funded much of the early work on this effort, HMO accreditation may ultimately achieve the same high standard as that used for hospitals. In fact, some employers now require that a plan have NCQA accreditation before they offer it to employees.

The Joint Commission on Accreditation of Healthcare Organizations, the organization best known for accrediting hospitals, began accrediting "networks" in 1994. Network accreditation focuses on the following key performance areas:

1. Preventive care.
2. The continuum of care.
3. The credentialing and performance of doctors, nurses, and other staff.
4. The rights of patients.
5. The procedures in place for measuring and improving the quality of patient care.
6. Education and communication.
7. Network leadership.
8. Management of information.

The Joint Commission examines services provided by

networks through ambulatory settings, home care, hospitals, laboratories, long-term care, and mental health.

Tip

To determine if an HMO is federally qualified, call the Health Care Financing Administration.

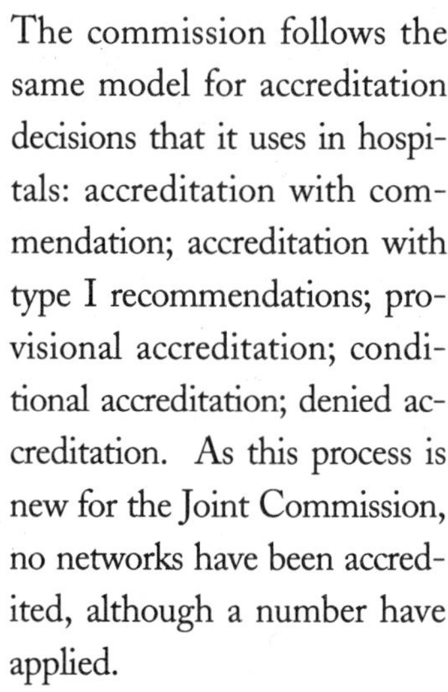

The commission follows the same model for accreditation decisions that it uses in hospitals: accreditation with commendation; accreditation with type I recommendations; provisional accreditation; conditional accreditation; denied accreditation. As this process is new for the Joint Commission, no networks have been accredited, although a number have applied.

Federal Government Qualification

Not quite the same as accreditation but a similar process, is that of federal qualification. HMOs that are federally qualified have been judged by the Office of Managed Care of the Health Care Financing Administration (HCFA) to meet certain basic standards of operation. An HMO must apply for qualification to the HCFA, which then visits the facility and considers such factors as health services delivery, availability, accessibility, quality assurance, financial stability, and marketing procedures before granting qualification. Qualification, which may take several months, is a one-time process unless an HMO is not initially approved and wishes to apply for approval at a later date. HMOs that are qualified are not subject to requalification. Hence, it is a good idea to find out how long an HMO has been federally qualified. The more recent the qualification, the better the chances that the HMO is still up to par.

To check on an HMO's accreditation, call the Joint Commission for the Accreditation of Healthcare Organizations or the National Committee for Quality Assurance (see Appendix L). To determine if an HMO is federally qualified, call the Health Care Financing Administration (see Appendix N).

Do Structure/Operation Make a Difference?

HMOs' organization and operating policies differ greatly, and the differences are not limited to type or model. HMOs typically offer a variety of plans, and each plan within that HMO can differ, not only on coverage but in its operating style.

The following is a list of issues and questions you should explore and answer when assessing an HMO. They address the question of how well the HMO can deliver quality care. If you are considering a number of HMOs, make copies of this list so that you have one for each plan you are considering. Having all the pertinent details will make it easier to compare the factors that are most important to you and your family and, thereby, choose the plan that suits you best.

Doctors/Other Staff

- Is there a sufficient number of primary care doctors from which to choose and are they accessible to you?
- What are the qualifications of the plan's doctors?

What percentage are board-certified? (Seek a minimum of 70 percent and preferably higher.)

- Can you choose your primary care doctor or are you assigned one? Can you change if you wish? How difficult is it?
- How long have the doctors been working for the plan? Has there been frequent turnover? If so, why?
- Are you given or can you request a list of the plan's doctors with information on their education and training?
- Are the doctors in whom you are interested still accepting patients? Are they pleased with the HMO and planning to continue the relationship?
- Do others besides your primary physician, such as nurse practitioners or physician's assistants, handle routine visits and examinations?
- Must you use only those specialists affiliated with the plan? Can you get a second opinion within the plan or go outside the plan for a second opinion?
- If the plan is affiliated with a teaching hospital, are medical students or residents involved in your care? If so, are you informed when a health professional is a student or resident?
- Is your primary physician involved in your care if you are hospitalized?
- If it is an IPA model, are the doctors you would select relatively close by?
- What provisions, if any, are made for evening, weekend, and emergency care?

- What provisions, if any, are made for care when you are away from home?
- If you don't like your doctor, what is the procedure for changing?

Hospitals

- Does the managed care plan utilize more than one hospital?
- What is the quality and scope of services offered? Do they have tertiary services such as burn care, open-heart surgery?
- Are the hospitals relatively close by and readily accessible?

Administration/Procedures

- How do you go about making an appointment?
- What are the procedures for referrals to specialists and subspecialists? Are there restrictions? What are they? Are the specialists you wish to see available to you?
- How will any preexisting conditions and illnesses be handled, financially and medically?
- If you change health plans during the course of treatment, or while pregnant, can you stay with your current doctor until the treatment is completed?
- Conversely, if your doctor leaves the plan, is he or she obligated to complete a course of treatment?
- What is the procedure for entering the hospital? How and when do you have to notify on an emergency/non-emergency basis?

- Is there a formulary (list of approved drugs)? Are generic substitutions made? Is it a restricted formulary in which substitutions are made as a matter of course with a blanket authorization from participating doctors?
- What kind of informational material does the managed care plan distribute to members?
- Is there a process for making an appeal if care has been denied, such as tests, medical or surgical procedures, second opinions?
- What is the procedure for seeking a second opinion outside of the plan?
- What are the procedures for staying with the plan if you leave your job but want to stay enrolled? Is that option available?

Services

- How long do you have to wait to get an appointment for a checkup or for treatment of a specific problem? If you have an appointment, how long will you usually wait to see the doctor?
- Does the managed care plan have central X-ray, laboratory, and pharmacy facilities? If not, where are these facilities located?
- Does the plan have a full range of health promotion programs, such as nutrition, exercise classes and health education?
- What health services are NOT provided by the plan?
- What happens if you receive care outside of the plan's area? What documents must you submit

and how long will you have to wait for reimbursement?

- What kind of grievance procedure does the plan have? How many complaints were filed in the last year and what were they about? How were those complaints resolved?
- How do you leave the plan if you wish to? Do you have to wait a year to drop out? Will you be given your medical records if you leave, or can you arrange for them to be transferred to another doctor?
- Can you join the plan if you are self-employed or must you belong to a group? Must you undergo a physical examination first and, if so, under what conditions can you be denied membership? Are there any conditions under which the plan can drop you from membership after you have joined?
- Which hospitals are affiliated with the plan? Are you expected to use the emergency rooms of these hospitals in a crisis or is there a 24-hour emergency center? What happens if you go to another hospital?

Outcomes

The last area we will describe for assessing the quality of managed care programs is an examination of outcomes. Outcomes is an old term that has a popular new use. It may seem obvious and overly simplistic, but outcomes are the results of care or treatments.

Most people assume that the outcomes of all kinds of care and treatment, including drugs and treatments, have been well studied. In a sense they have. The Food and Drug Administration (FDA) is responsible for the oversight of drugs and medical devices. However, once a drug is approved by the FDA as safe and efficacious (that it does what it's intended to do) there is very little follow-up on the use of drugs, devices, and treatments, especially as compared with others designed to achieve the same purpose. In fact, once drugs and devices are approved by the FDA, doctors have the right to use them as they see fit, even if that specific use has not been approved.

Satisfaction Measures in HMOs

Many HMOs do satisfaction surveys of their members. Following are examples of the kinds of ratings that are released to the public from these surveys:

- *Overall satisfaction ratings by their members.*
- *Ratings of doctors(as a group) by enrollees.*
- *HMO's responsiveness to complaints.*
- *Selection or choice of doctors.*

Outcomes studies could answer many important questions. For example, in some communities we know the cesarean section rate is two to three times that in other communities. What accounts for the discrepancy and what are the outcomes for mothers and babies? Or, for men with a particular stage of prostate cancer, what is better, surgery or radiotherapy? Outcomes studies will help determine the answers to these questions. The answers will help in the development of practice guidelines or practice parameters to guide doctors, hospitals, and HMOs in providing the best care possible. Outcomes studies are "in" today, and to their credit, HMOs have been leaders in this new field.

There is very little in the way of outcomes data available to the public on the results of care delivered by individual doctors and hospitals. The HCFA Medicare mortality studies described in Chapter 8 are an exception, as are the studies of mortality rates for patients undergoing coronary artery bypass surgery in New York State, where the State Health Department published the rates for individual physicians and hospitals. The movement is clearly in that direction, however, and in the years to come more report cards on how doctors, hospitals, and HMOs actually perform will emerge.

Tip

Report cards are now available for some HMOs. Ask HMOs you are considering what they have in outcome studies.

One leadership effort taking place under the aegis of the NCQA is the development of the Health Plan Employer Data Information Set (HEDIS 2.0). HEDIS 2.0 is the second refinement of a core set of performance measures that employers can use to understand what value their health care dollars are purchasing. The HEDIS performance measures can also serve as a standard of accountability for HMOs. NCQA is providing the leadership and working with employers and providers in the development of HEDIS.

Many large employers are requesting HEDIS data from managed care plans. As many as half of the nation's managed care plans have already received requests for data from employers. A few employers have given HEDIS data, in some modified fashion, to employees so they can use it in making their selections of managed care plans.

In the coming years it is likely that more employers and managed care plans will release report cards based on HEDIS data to employees and to the public. If you work for a large company, you should ask your human resources department about HEDIS 2.0 and if data derived from it can be made available to you.

Report cards are already available for some HMOs, and those HMOs are leading the trend in disclosing outcomes measures. Kaiser-Permanente, United Health Care, and US Health Care have all published their version of a report card. Listed below are some of the things you can find out from these report cards, or from other data maintained by HMOs.

Ask the HMO or the state insurance or health department for these studies and use them to compare managed care programs.

If an HMO you are considering does not have or is not willing to share this kind of data, ask instead about the transfer or dropout rate. In many states, HMOs are required to maintain a record of those who leave the plan each year, usually noted as a percentage of total enrollment. If that number is too high compared with other HMOs in the region, it may be a good indication of dissatisfied enrollees. As the saying goes, "people vote with their feet."

In the Washington, DC area and in a few other areas, the magazine *Health Pages* reports this kind of information on HMOs in the region.

Only a few, relatively large, HMOs are actively engaged in measuring and sharing the results of outcomes studies. A survey by A. Foster Higgins Co., reported in *Business & Health* magazine, showed 26 percent of HMOs conducted no outcomes studies and 44 percent were "somewhat active." Yet, the work of a few leaders, and that of groups such as the Health Outcomes Institute, a not-for-profit entity established in 1993 to develop and distribute the Outcomes Management System, can be a model for others. As indicated by its name, the mission of the Health Outcomes Institute is to encourage the development and dissemination of public domain tools and techniques for measuring the effectiveness of health care.

Even HMOs that do not issue report cards still may have some of the outcomes data described in the following pages and may be willing to release it if requested. In some states, health departments may require this or similar data, and you may be able to get it from the state health department. In the absence of outcomes data you must make quality judgements based on accreditation and process and structure, but you should try to obtain outcomes data whenever possible.

Following are examples of the kinds of outcomes data reported by HMOs. These were excerpted from a report, "Quality Report Card," by one of the nation's leading HMOs, Kaiser Permanente of Northern California. It is difficult to make judgements on these measures in the abstract, so usually the HMO provides companion data as a standard or benchmark.

	Reported result	*Benchmark*
Immunization of children (higher is better)	93.2%	45.1%
Mammography screening rate (higher is better)	71.2%	—
Flu shots for adults (higher is better)	57.6%	46.0%
Annual retinal exam for diabetics (higher is better)	51.0%	—
Laminectomy (removal of a spinal disc) rate (lower is better)	47.2%	91.7%
Cesarean delivery rate (lower is better)	16.1%	22.5%
Vaginal birth after cesarean (higher is better)	50.7%	—
Perinatal mortality (deaths at birth or within the first few days after birth) rate (lower is better)	8.7%	9.5%
Hypertension screening rate (higher is better)	93.1%	—
Appendix rupture rate (lower is better)	23.8%	29.0%
Outpatient follow-up after inpatient discharge for major affective disorder (higher is better)	70.0%	—

Not all of this data is available from most HMOs. In fact, many fall woefully short of any useful data to judge quality. But ask. The better the information you receive, the more interested the HMO is in quality care and good communications with its members.

Additional Checks on the Quality of HMOs

Complaint ratios

In many states, HMOs, or state health or insurance departments, maintain a log of complaints. Try to get the number of complaints filed and divide by the number of enrollees. This will give you a ratio of complaints per enrollee. (The New York City Department of Consumer Affairs identified complaint ratios ranging from 116 enrollees per complaint to 1,910 enrollees per complaint in a study they conducted of HMOs.)

Tip

In the coming years it is likely that more employers and managed care plans will release "report cards" based on HEDIS data to employees and to the public. If you work for a large company, you should ask your human resources department about HEDIS 2.0 and if data derived from it can be made available to you.

Dropout rate

It is possible, in some states, to find out from an HMO, or from the insurance or health departments, the number of enrollees who left the plan during a year. Get that figure and divide it by the total enrollment and multiply it by 100 to get the dropout percentage. If the rate is higher than for other HMOs, it probably indicates enrollee dissatisfaction. (A review by *Consumers' Checkbook* showed "quit ranges" of 3 percent to 25 percent for a group of more than a dozen HMOs they reviewed.)

Enrollment figures

Ideally, there is a relationship between quality and success. Based on this assumption, a high-quality, successful HMO should be growing, as lesser-quality, less successful HMOs are declining in enrollment-although other factors come into play. Ask the HMO for its enrollment history for at least the past three years.

HMO Doctors: The Rules are Different, Is the Care as Good?

Chapter 18

Many people question the quality of doctors associated with HMOs. In some cases, especially when a plan first enters a particular region, it may sign up virtually any licensed doctor who applies. At the same time, many plans have rigorous selection standards and state correctly that they screen their doctors carefully, while any doctor with a license can hang up a shingle and practice in the community.

It is important to point out that doctors seeking new patients are not necessarily poor doctors. They may simply be new to an area, establishing a new practice arrangement, or be recently trained and beginning a practice. What seems to happen, however, is that when an HMO achieves a significant market penetration and begins to control the flow of large numbers of patients, more doctors sign on. Also, many hospitals encourage their doctors to sign on with as many different plans as possible in order to insure that the hospital does not lose any potential patients. In fact, over 70 percent of all doctors participate in at least one managed care arrangement.

Over 70 percent of all doctors participate in at least one managed care arrangement.

The main factor to focus on in assessing an HMO is its resources, primarily doctors and hospitals. First, is there an ample selection of primary care doctors near where you live and work? Second, are the doctors well qualified? This can be answered by following the approach outlined in this book for finding the best doctors. When choosing doctors, it is usually a good idea to call their offices to confirm they are still affiliated with the particular plan. Some HMOs have been known to pad their panels by continuing to list doctors who are no longer with them or who don't accept new patients. Also, it is a good idea to check on the procedure for using the doctor listed.

Tip

Unlike indemnity plans in which you can find a specialist on your own if you choose, in managed care plans, you must be referred to see a specialist.

HMOs may list hundreds of doctors but not all of them are necessarily accessible. A large HMO, for example, may restrict the number of specialists that primary care doctors can refer to for various reasons, including location, hospital capacity, and general resource allocation. So although you may see the name of an ophthalmologist, gynecologist, or other specialist you want to use, and indeed that doctor may be affiliated with the HMO, it does not necessarily follow that your primary care doctor is free to refer you to them. Those specialists may see HMO patients only on a certain basis—for specific procedures, for example, or in a certain geographic region—and then possibly only after a rigorous screening process. These possibilities illustrate the varying styles of operation you will find in managed care plans.

One important note: Doctors in HMOs are bound by the same professional ethics that guide all doctors. However, there is a major difference: In an HMO, the plan is responsible for providing you with care as well as with a doctor. If your doctor leaves the plan, you don't follow him or her. The plan provides a new doctor for you.

Selecting Doctors in an HMO

Selecting a doctor in an HMO can be a greater challenge than selecting one when you have indemnity insurance that leaves you free to select a doctor without the restrictions of the plan. Obviously, in an HMO arrangement you need to select a doctor who belongs to that plan. Studies have shown that about 40 percent of enrollees in managed care plans have to choose a new doctor when they join. However, even in a plan of small size, you will usually have the option of choosing among a number of primary care doctors as well as other specialists and subspecialists. In doing so, utilize the same criteria you would apply to selecting a doctor in a fee-for-service practice.

According to a 1993 study by the National Research Corporation, a higher percentage of participants in HMOs say they are more satisfied with their health plans than those who have traditional indemnity plans or are in a preferred-provider organization.

The first doctor you select in an HMO plan is your primary care doctor. Typically, you will be sent a list with little information other than the doctor's name, specialty, and address. *Find out more about those doctors you may be considering.* Use the process described in Section I to guide you.

If you make a selection and are not satisfied, request a change. Ask about the procedure before you join the plan.

Some critics observe that in fee-for-service medicine the doctor has a financial incentive to provide more rather than less care, even if it is not necessary, and that such practices contribute to increasing health care costs.

When you need a specialist, it is your primary care doctor who will refer you, as in traditional indemnity plans. But, unlike indemnity plans in which you can find a specialist on your own if you choose, in managed care plans, you must be referred to see a specialist. Again, your choices will be limited in selecting specialists, but be assertive. Ask for a choice of doctors and ask why your primary care doctor recommends a particular specialist. One disadvantage to the HMO model and the network referral process is that primary care doctors can end up making referrals to specialists and/or subspecialists they do not know. This may result in poor communication between the primary care doctor and the specialists, which is not in the patient's best interest. If you are not satisfied with the choices offered, ask to go outside the plan. Choice of providers outside a plan is built into a POS plan and is permitted in many others under certain conditions.

However, if you do not have a choice, or if the choices are not ones with which you agree, consider going outside the HMO. Although you are likely to have to pay more, it may be worth it if you get a correct diagnosis and appropriate treatment for your problem. In some cases, the HMO will agree to pay at least a consultation fee if you feel strongly that you need to discuss your problem with another doctor. After the consultation, if you still feel the need for a different doctor, at least your choice will be based on more complete information.

How Doctors and Patients Feel about Managed Care

A recent study of more than 1,700 patients reported in the *Journal of the American Medical Association (JAMA)* found widespread dissatisfaction with HMOs and other managed care plans. Patients reported that independent doctors were easier to contact by telephone, more willing to schedule office appointments on short notice, and showed more interest in their well-being than doctors associated with HMOs.

A 1992 Consumer Reports *survey of patient response to HMOs demonstrated that members were more satisfied with plans that paid their doctor on a fee basis than they were with those that paid on a capitated, or per-person, basis.*

On the other hand, according to a 1993 study by the National Research Corporation, a higher percentage of participants in HMOs say they are more satisfied with their health plans than those who have traditional indemnity plans or are in a preferred-provider organization. The positive ratings reflected in this study are reinforced by the research conducted by the Novalis Research Group, which said that 85 percent of HMO members rated the quality of their health services "excellent" or "good."

Tip

Doctors in HMOs are bound by the same professional ethics that guide all doctors. However, there is a major difference: In an HMO, the plan is responsible for providing you with care as well as with a doctor. If your doctor leaves the plan, you don't follow him or her. The plan provides a new doctor for you.

With results somewhere in between is a 1992 *Consumer Reports* survey of patient response to HMOs which demonstrated that members were more satisfied with plans that paid their doctor on a fee basis than they were with those that paid on a capitated, or per-person, basis.

In certain instances, capitation arrangements may place the insurance burden on the doctor or medical group. For example, groups of obstetricians and gynecologists may be paid a fixed, general fee per person to provide all appropriate services to a group of 1,000 women. Both the insurer and the doctor group have formed estimates about the services necessary, based on the demographics of the group (age, education, income, work status, etc.). Both groups would anticipate that a certain number of births, hysterectomies, vaginal cancers, etc., would occur within the total population. The doctor group then assumes the risk that the total fee will reimburse them appropriately. If their projections are wrong and many more services are required, then they could suffer financial loss.

Some doctors have complaints about HMOs. While the paperwork is reduced for patients, it may be increased for doctors, especially in the IPA model. HMOs impose and enforce strict controls on doctors by closely monitoring care, tests, and prescriptions. Doctors who exceed these limits ("outliers") may be dropped or disciplined. This process of measuring the costs of care provided by a doctor is known to those on the inside as "economic credentialing." The plans monitor much of this through reviews and case management techniques, which often require a great many reports from doctors. All the additional paperwork required by insurers and regulators, both in managed care and in indemnity plans, reduces the time doctors are able to spend with patients.

Tip

In some cases, the HMO will agree to pay at least a consultation fee if you feel strongly that you need to discuss your problem with another doctor. Do not hesitate to ask.

Doctors also frequently complain that when a plan gains a firm foothold in a market and controls significant patient flow, it uses its bargaining power to reduce doctors' fees. Of course, that is exactly the approach many health policy experts encourage as a way to reduce costs!

Another concern expressed by some observers is the amount of money many for-profit HMOs spend in marketing their plans to the public through advertising and public relations campaigns. As in the case of for-profit hospitals, some critics are troubled that a substantial portion of an organization's income may be used for these purposes, which are not directly patient-related. It is estimated that for-profit HMOs spend 69 to 70 cents of every dollar on care while not-for-profits spend 96 to 97 cents.

Many doctors have begun to encounter exclusion from managed care networks. These doctors have sued the HMOs, claiming that they should be included in the doctor panels or lists if they are willing to abide by the fees and procedures set by the HMO. The legal actions—called "willing provider" lawsuits—have become a major issue at local, state, and national levels.

The Payment Factor

Doctors in HMOs may be paid in a number of ways, and the method seems to have an influence on patient satisfaction. The three primary methods are fee-for-service, but typically with negotiated fees; capitation, in which a provider (hospital, doctor, etc.) is paid a set amount per person to provide all care; and salary. In a survey of HMOs by a Washington consumers' group, respondents felt that doctors who were paid salaries spent more time with patients than those compensated in other ways.

All the additional paperwork required by insurers and regulators, both in managed care and in indemnity plans, reduces the time doctors are able to spend with patients.

Some people are troubled by the shifting of doctor incentives in various kinds of HMOs. In traditional fee-for-service medicine the doctor is paid a fee for every procedure performed. As a result, the doctor has little incentive—other than professional ethics—to restrict the amount and cost of care delivered. Indeed, some critics observe that in fee-for-service medicine the doctor has a financial incentive to provide more rather than less care, even if it is not necessary, and that such practices contribute to increasing health care costs.

On the other hand, critics of HMOs contend that doctors in some of these practice arrangements may have incentives to provide fewer services, even if more are justified. This is referred to as "bedside rationing." It is a particular concern if the doctor is financially penalized for ordering too many tests, or too frequently referring patients to specialists, and budgets are exceeded. It also troubles people that doctors may be financially rewarded if, for example, no referrals are made or certain tests are not prescribed. Both of these practices now occur in certain HMOs. In such instances, critics want to know, who is looking out for the patient's best interests? Supporters of HMOs respond by pointing to the overall financial penalties if a patient's illness is allowed to spiral, leading to expensive hospitalization.

Critics of HMOs contend that doctors in some of these practice arrangements may have incentives to provide fewer services, even if more are justified.

Although supporters insist that this cost threat serves as a built-in check to assure effective patient care, some dissatisfied members of HMOs would disagree. Advocates of HMOs also argue that these organizations monitor doctors' practice patterns carefully, not just to control costs but also to assess the quality of care. While it is true that in order to control costs an HMO must restrict access to health care services such as doctors, drugs, hospitalizations, and procedures, the theory is that what will be cut out is the waste in the system and not necessary care. Most studies have shown that enrollees in HMOs use about the same amount of health care resources at about the same rate as people not enrolled in HMOs, with the exception of hospital days, which HMOs reduce by about 30 percent.

Most studies have shown that enrollees in HMOs use about the same amount of health care resources at about the same rate as people not enrolled in HMOs, with the exception of hospital days, which HMOs reduce by about 30 percent.

Charges vs. Fee Schedule

When discussing charges you pay, especially for service outside the HMO network, always clarify the differences between charges and fee schedules. For example:

- *If an HMO states it covers 90 percent of a fee, is it 90 percent of what the doctor charges or 90 percent of an approved or allowable fee schedule?*

  A doctor may bill you $1,000 for a procedure but the HMO may have an allowable charge of only $500. Is the HMO willing to pay 90 percent of $1,000 or 90 percent of $500?

  (This is important to know for all insurance, indemnity or HMOs.) "Out of network" charges are usually substantially higher.

- *It is important with HMOs, as it is with any insurer, to follow the organization's procedures for arranging medical care and paying for it. HMOs have procedures in place for administrating these two important aspects of their operation, and controlling costs is one of the major goals. Courts have upheld an HMO's right to refuse to pay healthcare costs if these procedures have not been followed.*

- *Remember, HMOs are insurers as well as providers and have rights and responsibilities similar to other insurers.*

How to Join an HMO

Chapter 19

Any employer with at least 25 employees that provides a health plan for employees, and is not self-insured, must offer one or more HMOs as alternatives to the traditional health insurance program it offers. If your employer pays all or a portion of the cost of a traditional health plan for you, he must make at least the same contribution to the cost of an HMO.

There is usually an open enrollment period once a year, during which time you have the opportunity to choose health insurance or an HMO. If you become dissatisfied with your choice, you generally cannot drop out until the next enrollment period a year later. To join an HMO you must live in its service area—a geographic area that serves the plan's membership.

If you become a member and later leave your employer, you generally can convert to individual membership without furnishing evidence of insurability. Some HMOs will accept you as a member if you are self-employed, but they may require you to undergo a physical examination first.

When you reach age 65 and become eligible for Medicare, you can continue to receive your medical care from the plan if it has a contract with Medicare. You will have to pay the monthly Medicare Part B premium and, most likely, a monthly premium.

If you are still working when you reach age 65 and have been enrolled in an HMO through your employer, you may continue to use the plan as your primary health coverage. Medicare will reimburse you only for medical care that is not provided through your plan but which is covered by Medicare.

Tip

If you become a member and later leave your employer, you generally can convert to individual membership without furnishing evidence of insurability.

If you keep working past age 65, you have the same rights as younger employees to select an HMO at the next open enrollment. You also have the option at age 65 to choose Medicare as your primary health coverage. Under such circumstances, you may elect to receive your Medicare benefits from a plan as described above.

If you are planning to continue to work after age 65 you should visit your local Social Security office for information about health coverage options.

The Group Health Association of America and the American Association of Retired Persons have developed a joint guide for choosing HMOs that may also be helpful to the older person (see Appendix L).

Section Four

Cost, Quality, and Consumers:

You Can Cut Your Health Care Costs.

Here's How.

Key Terms

▼ Consumer Price Index (CPI)

A statistic produced by the federal government to measure inflation. The CPI compares the price of certain goods and services at a given date against the average price for the same goods and services at a reference date.

▼ Cost Shifting

The practice by health insurance providers of increasing the charges to one group of patients (such as private pay patients, who presumably have the ability to pay) when the payment for another group of patients will not cover the costs for that group. For example, individuals with insurance ultimately bear the cost for those without insurance.

▼ Rationing

The practice of making certain expensive health care procedures, such as transplants or cardiac catheterizations, available in limited numbers.

Is There a Health Care Crisis: If So, How Does it Affect You?

Chapter 20

The concern about a "health care crisis," like many other issues, is in the eye of the beholder. To employers paying rapidly escalating health care insurance rates, there may be a crisis. To a family with no insurance and large health bills, there may be a crisis. To the family whose primary breadwinner has lost not only a job but health insurance, there may be a crisis. On the other hand, the potential of reform, and a new system of health care insurance, may be a crisis to small business owners who could be driven out of business if they have to buy health insurance for their employees. Or a crisis may exist for the insurance agents or insurance companies that could see their businesses devastated if certain kinds of reform are adopted. But for someone who has a good health insurance plan, paid for by an employer, the crisis may be, in fact, no crisis.

So whether a crisis does or does not exist depends on your perception. While there may not be agreement on the definition and existence of a crisis, what is clear is that many Americans agree that certain aspects of our health care system need to be changed—although there is little agreement on who should pay for the changes and how. Three things prompt this widely shared belief:

Cost

Most Americans, especially those who pay the bills

for health care, believe costs are out of control. Medical inflation has topped the overall inflation rate since 1981. Health care now consumes almost 15 percent of our GDP (gross domestic product) as compared with only 7.4 percent in 1970. Currently, our nation spends about $1 trillion on health care, and some estimates project $2 trillion by the year 2000. That will amount to about $14,500 for a family as compared with about $7,700 today. It would also account for about 20 percent of the total US economy as compared with 7.4 percent in 1970.

Access

Access to most people not only means access to health care, but to doctors, hospitals, and health plans of *their* choice. While many are willing to have their options limited to some degree, they do not want to entirely lose their right to choose providers.

Also, most Americans want security in health care. That is, if they lose their jobs they still want some type of "safety net." Even if unemployed, they want access to health care without it being financially devastating.

If there is a major health care reform, Americans are concerned that quality and choice may be diminished.

There is a concern shared by many Americans that too many people lack access to good health care because they lack insurance. In fact, some 37.4 million of the US population are without health insurance at some time during a one-year period, and many others are fearful that if they lost their jobs, they, and their families, would join the ranks of the uninsured. Even those without insurance still receive care, but it is sporadic and expensive and all those who pay for health insurance bear the cost of this care in a process known as "cost shifting."

Quality

Quality is another highly esteemed value in health care. When someone inquires about obtaining health care, they do not ask for the cheapest care. They ask for the best care! In theory Americans may acknowledge the need for limits, but when it comes to themselves and their families, they want the best and they want it without limitation. That is why the "R" word, rationing, is not frequently heard in the debates on health care reform.

Most Americans believe the care they receive is of good quality, but they are concerned about two aspects of it. First, if there is major health care reform, particularly if elements of managed care are incorporated, will quality be diminished? (They are also concerned that choice may be diminished.) Second, a question that concerns policymakers more than the ordinary citizen, is whether the quality we receive as a nation is worth the price we pay. Although we spend more money per capita on health care than any other nation, we rank only 18th in life expectancy, one important measure of a population's health.

To most Americans, access not only means access to health care, but to doctors, hospitals, and health plans of their choice.

There are other factors that fuel the issue, and the general perception is one of a health care system in need of change. Clearly, our nation's political leadership is responding in that fashion. Included among the factors prompting this new attitude are the costs of malpractice, the overabundance of medical specialists, the paperwork burden, and the fraud and waste inherent in our present system (the latter alone is estimated by some to cost $200 billion). But the heart of the matter lies in the basic issues of cost, access, and quality.

Many Americans have come to believe that health care is a right, not a privilege. And, as a right, they expect someone else, whether it is the government or their employer, to ensure that right and to pay for most of it.

In reality, the direct financial burden placed on most American families as a result of health care expenditures has decreased significantly in recent decades. The direct costs and the major burden of paying for health care have been shifted from patients to private employers and the government. In 1960 patients paid 48 percent of all medical bills while in 1993 they paid only 21 percent. Also, according to the US Bureau of Health Statistics, as a share of direct household spending, health care expenses actually fell 40 percent between 1960 and 1988.

Private business pays 51.7 percent of the nation's health care bills. And government spending has the same upward spiral.

At the same time, the costs to employers and the government have increased relatively and absolutely. For example, private business now pays 51.7 percent of the nation's health care bills. And government spending has the same upward spiral. When conceived in 1965, the cost for Medicare in 1990 was projected to be $9 billion. It was actually $106 billion in 1990. Similarly, Medicaid, when created in 1965, was projected at $1 billion in 1990, but the actual bill was $76 billion. Of course, we all ultimately share that bill, directly and indirectly, through taxes and deferred wages.

Americans are proud of their health care system, even while recognizing its weaknesses. They do not want to diminish its strengths, only to strengthen its weaknesses.

In 1994, a new trend emerged. The rate of increase in health care costs began to slow. The consumer price index for medical care rose only 4.9 percent from February 1993 to February 1994, the lowest increase in a decade. One of the primary reasons for the slow-down in cost is that those who directly pay for health care, employers and government, either independently or in coalitions, have become smarter, more aggressive buyers. In addition, managed care has brought intensive competition to the health care market. These trends have forced traditional providers, especially doctors and hospitals, to bargain and to compete for patients and for market share. All of this has brought more of a true market mentality (sellers competing for buyers by offering the best price, quality, and service) to health care.

Whatever form our health care system takes in the near future, either as a result of market forces or legislation, will, of necessity, be based on the values Americans hold on health care. Americans are proud of their health care system, even while recognizing its weaknesses. They do not want to diminish its strengths, only to strengthen its weaknesses.

Doctors' Fees: a Prime Target

Doctors' fees are among the most controversial aspects of health care. Doctors are a favorite target of health care critics, and there seems to be a lack of sympathy for them from politicians and a large segment of the public.

While compensation levels for some doctors are probably too high, others are clearly too low. Fees for some procedures that have been made faster and simpler by new technology, and require much less of a doctor's time, are probably too high, while compensation for nontechnical patient care, usually involving considerable face-to-face time, is definitely too low.

The following questions should be answered early on in the first office visit.

- *Are fees reasonable relative to those charged by other doctors for the same or similar services?*
- *Is the fee covered in total or in part by medical insurance?*

The long-running argument over doctors' incomes and, indeed, over costs in health care does not seem important when it comes to an individual or family attempting to establish a relationship with a doctor. We all want the best. What you as a consumer should be most concerned with is not paying more than you have to, even while you strive to get the best care.

Patients should not feel uncomfortable about raising the issue of fees, and most doctors will discuss them willingly. In the best-case situation, the doctor should open the discussion of fees for a specific procedure before it takes place—especially since it is not uncommon for many doctors to require payment first, expecting the patient to be reimbursed later. Since many doctors now accept less than "usual and customary" fees from managed care organizations, it is not inappropriate to ask a doctor if he or she will charge you the same fee as an HMO patient would pay. Many will.

The simplest and most effective way to check on the relative price, or fee, is to talk with a number of doctors as well as your insurance carrier. Insurance companies typically have set fees for specific procedures and services. These will guide you not only in relative pricing, but also in what portion you will bear if your insurance does not cover the total cost.

Your Role in the Health Cost Debate

Chapter 21

Despite its overwhelming complexity, it is possible for the individual consumer to play a role in helping to solve our nation's health cost problem. Although it is often difficult to gauge the impact of an individual action, collectively we all make up an important part of the health care market, as consumers, or purchasers, of health care. Together, our behavior as consumers adds up to the demand side of the health care equation, a very important factor in determining price, supply, and quality.

In the health care market, when someone else, usually an employer or the government, pays most of the bill, we often do not behave as responsible consumers. But when it's money out of our own pockets, our behavior changes.

The first and most important thing we can do is behave as consumers. In the health care market, when someone else, usually an employer or the government, pays most of the bill, we often do not behave as responsible consumers. But when it's money out of our own pockets, our behavior changes. Ultimately, however, it *is* money out of our pockets, either through more taxes or reduced wages, so it behooves us all to approach health care with a true consumer mentality by making certain all the health care we receive is necessary and worth the price.

Six Tips for Smart Health Care Consumers

Don't use health care resources unnecessarily

Remember, ultimately you do pay. Don't demand additional tests or treatments solely for reassurance if your doctor does not recommend them. Of course, if you feel your problem has not been identified or treated properly, that is another issue. On the other hand, a doctor may recommend diagnostic tests in the mistaken belief that you want them. You should question any procedures that you feel are unnecessary. In using health care resources judiciously, be aware that hospitalization costs make up the largest portion of our national health bill (close to 40 percent). At one time in our history, doctors and patients looked with favor on inpatient care. That was the only way people could be reimbursed by health insurance. That has changed, and care that is delivered on an outpatient or ambulatory basis, or at home, can be of high quality and cost-effective.

Engage in a healthy lifestyle

Behavior and habits that keep you healthy reduce your need for health care. Excessive drinking, smoking, obesity, and other risky behaviors substantially increase our health costs. A recent study in the *New England Journal of Medicine* showed that, based on health habits, those with low risk had average claims of $190 over three years while those at high risk had claims averaging $1,550 over three years. Another study reported in *Managed Health Care* estimated that 24 percent of hospital admissions were related to lifestyle. Alcohol and drug abuse, for example, are estimated to cost our economy over $150 billion in direct health costs and in related costs such as lost productivity and premature death. Violence, according to the National Public Services Research Institute, adds some $15.5 billion to our nation's health care bill. Smoking, according to the Centers for Disease Control and Prevention, adds another $50 billion annually.

Comparison shop

Look for the best quality at the best price. Poor quality health care is the most expensive health care. Make certain your health care providers and the health care you receive are of good quality. Also, make certain the prices you are charged are comparable with what other providers charge. Don't be embarrassed to ask about fees and prices and don't be shy about comparison shopping.

> *Tip*
>
> *Poor quality health care is the most expensive health care.*

Study your coverages

If you are in an HMO, and especially if you are in an indemnity plan, make certain you are reimbursed properly for your bills.

Make certain your medical bills are accurate

Medical bills frequently contain errors. Read them carefully, not only to be sure you receive proper reimbursement, but also to be certain the charges are correct. Even though your insurance company or HMO may foot the bill, ultimately, you will pay for it.

Be a knowledgeable consumer

You should understand not only your own health care plan but also what reforms are being proposed on the national level. Express your opinions and concerns to your elected state and federal representatives. The opinions of individual voters do make a difference and, like every other national issue, special interest groups do try to influence legislation to their benefit. However, the largest special-interest group is voters, and elected officials do respond to voter concerns. Express yours.

How to Catch Costly Billing Errors

Chapter 22

A study from the federal General Accounting Office in Washington DC in 1991 found overcharges in as many as 95 percent of hospital bills.

Stories abound about such errors. Consider the case of the parents who received a bill for the circumcision of their newborn—a baby girl. Or the report of the man who had surgery to replace two of his heart valves with synthetic devices—and was charged for replacement of 200.

Most people take it for granted that their hospital bill is correct when, in fact, they might better assume the opposite.

These errors can just slip by unnoticed. For one thing, most people take it for granted that their hospital bill is correct when, in fact, they might better assume the opposite.

And even when they do find blatant errors, many patients are reluctant to question the doctor or hospital billing office for fear of repercussions.

If you have time to plan for a hospital stay, there are steps you can take to head off bill errors even before they crop up:

- Talk about fees with the doctor and a patient representative at the hospital where you will be admitted to pin down what the charges will be. Then talk to your insurance representative to determine if all the charges will be covered. If not, ask the doctor to accept the insurance as payment in full. It costs nothing to ask and you could save money.

- Don't go to a doctor's office or hospital alone if you are anxious and fearful because it is likely that you will not understand or recall important information and instructions; it may help to have two sets of ears and eyes. And keep a written record of your office visit or hospital stay; no one knows better than you whether or not you received the services and medications listed on a bill.

- While you may have to pay as you leave a doctor's office, you should never settle a hospital bill as you leave. Insist that you be sent an itemized (not a summary) bill with descriptions of services, not just codes. And insist on your hospital records, too; it's the best way of comparing what was done to you with what your bill says was done to you. Inform the hospital's billing department that you want to verify your bill before it is submitted to your insurance provider. You may meet with resistance since hospitals want to get paid as fast as possible, but don't give in. You need time to review the bill, which is usually a document of substantial size and detail.

Tip

Talk about fees with the doctor and a patient representative at the hospital where you will be admitted to pin down what the charges will be. Then talk to your insurance representative to determine if all the charges will be covered.

Here are some of the excesses that can slip onto medical bills:

Code errors

There are more than 7,000 five-digit codes for health services and procedures. A revised system went into effect in 1992; because it's still relatively new, doctors and other health care workers can make mistakes. And never accept a bill with only codes, because they tell you nothing. Your bill must also have understandable explanations so that you can make sure the codes correspond to what was done to you.

Tip

Keep a written record of your office visit or hospital stay; no one knows better than you whether or not you received the services and medications listed on a bill.

Duplicate billings

This happens with relatively minor items, such as urine and stool tests—all of which get buried amid the big billings such as high-tech tests.

Redundant or shoddy testing

If multiple doctors are involved in your care, each may request the same test. If you find yourself going through the same procedure, question it immediately. Also, you should refuse to pay for repeats of unclear X-rays and blood tests involving inadequate samples if they are the laboratory's fault.

Unauthorized charges

Certain routine tests, such as a chest X-ray, may be

done without your permission. If you have insisted on giving advance approval for all such expenses, don't pay for tests you haven't agreed to.

"Phantom" charges

Many hospitals have a standard list of fees that are automatically imposed in connection with certain procedures (for example, a charge for a sedative and other medication even when a child is delivered through natural childbirth). Demand removal of such charges as well as those related to tests that are canceled by your doctor.

Unrequested items

There are no freebies in hospitals. Personal items (for example, slippers, tissues, and toothpaste) may be billed at luxury rates. Look for and contest confusingly named items such as "thermal therapy kit: $15," which may be a plastic bag of ice cubes or "urinal: $5," which may be a plastic cup.

Bulk charges

Look for vague listings such as "pharmacy" or "radiology." Ask for an itemized listing and question anything that appears to be a charge over and above the total for specific items.

Unbundling

On the other hand, routine procedures may be broken down into separate parts, each charged separately. This kind of "creative billing" results in making the sum of the parts greater than the whole.

Human errors

A mistake in data entry can happen if a clerical worker is not paying strict attention. Hospitals call these "honest mistakes," but they don't try to correct them unless you insist.

If you find an error—or many—call the hospital billing department right away. Insist that the bill not be sent to your insurance carrier until it is straightened out; if it's already in the works, write to your insurer and report the discrepancy.

How to Get Insurers to Pay

Chapter 23

There are a number of justifiable reasons why insurers refuse to pay for care received. Many plans, for example, don't include dentistry and psychiatric treatment because such coverage would raise the company's cost for employees' coverage. Sometimes the treatment may occur before your effective date of coverage (there is usually a waiting period for pre-existing conditions). In other instances, the doctor's fee may be considered to be in excess of the usual, prevailing, and customary fees in the area, or the doctor may enter an incorrect code number for the procedure on the insurance claim form. Before getting up in arms over a denied claim, make sure you are actually entitled to it under the terms of your contract. If the error can be traced to your doctor, contact his or her office—in writing—and point out the discrepancy.

An Assertive Approach

If you believe the insurance company has made a mistake, try these tactics:

Write to a high official in the company with your appeal as soon as you receive the unsatisfactory explanation of benefits (EOB) form. The letter should summarize the elements of the dispute and contain your name and, if it is different, the name of the insured, the policy number, claim number, and copies (not originals) of any additional documents.

Write to your state insurance commissioner, enclosing copies of all correspondence between you and your insurer. Every state insurance department has a consumer complaint division that cannot order the insurer to pay you, but can certainly intercede on your behalf to make sure your appeal is considered promptly and seriously.

Tip

Every state insurance department has a consumer complaint division that can intercede on your behalf with insurance companies.

Bring legal action against the insurer. Depending on the amount, you can do this in small claims court on your own or consult a lawyer about a full-scale suit.

If you need advice or referrals call the National Insurance Consumer Helpline, which is sponsered by a number of insurance associations. The telephone number for the Helpline and for each state insurance department are listed in Appendix H.

Medical Flexible Spending Accounts

An excellent device for saving money on health care is the flexible spending account whereby employees may set aside pre-tax money each year. The total dollar amount you elect to set aside (the allowable amount varies by employer but may be up to $2,000) is broken out over the number of pay periods remaining in that year. Throughout the year, the money is deducted directly from your paycheck and put into an account.

When your request for medical reimbursement (to pay for deductibles, co-pays, dental care, prescriptions, etc.) is granted, you are personally reimbursed with your own, pre-tax money which is deducted from your account. You will not be taxed on this reimbursement but there is one catch: the money must be used within the calendar year or it is lost!

SECTION FIVE

Special Health Care Choices:

Consider the Needs of Women, Children, Older Adults, and Emergency Patients.

Here's How.

KEY TERMS

▼ **AUTOIMMUNE REACTION/DISEASES**
A response or illness in which a person produces an immune response to his or her own antigens, often resulting in the destruction of cells or organs.

▼ **CEREBROVASCULAR**
Relating to the blood supply to the brain.

▼ **DEFIBRILLATOR**
A machine designed to restore normal heartbeat through the use of electric shock.

▼ **DEMENTIA**
A general mental deterioration due to organic or psychological factors.

▼ **HUMAN PAPILLOMAVIRUS**
A family of viruses that manifest in benign, wart-like protrusions.

▼ **OSTEOPOROSIS**
A condition that results from a reduction in bone mass, osteoporosis commonly occurs in postmenopausal women and elderly men.

▼ **THORACIC**
Pertaining to the chest.

THE SPECIAL HEALTH CARE NEEDS OF WOMEN

CHAPTER 24

Women are America's major health care consumers, spending two out of every three dollars earmarked for health care, visiting health care providers 25 percent more often than men, and living longer than men. Because of this longer life span, the assumption is that women are healthier, when, in fact, women are affected with serious and debilitating diseases such as heart disease, diabetes, arthritis, stroke, and clinical depression, which confer a poorer quality of life, especially in later years.

A recent survey of American women's health by Louis Harris and Associates, sponsored by The Commonwealth Fund, a national philanthropic organization located in New York City, found major health care problems. Among them:

- Heart disease, which accounts for about 31 percent of female deaths, is the leading cause of death among American women as it is among American men. However, cancer and diabetes have been gaining on heart disease. The proportion of female deaths from these two causes increased in the past two years.
- Lung cancer has replaced breast cancer as the leading cause of women's deaths from cancer.
- Smoking rates are declining faster for women than for men, except among women in their childbearing years. More than 28 percent of women age 25 to 34 smoke cigarettes.

- Because women have a longer life expectancy than men (83 years vs. 76 years), they are more likely to acquire the diseases associated with very old age, including Alzheimer's and complications arising from osteoporosis.

Many experts believe that the health of women is harmed by medical specialization; indeed, many women must make the medical rounds to two and sometimes three doctors in order to ensure complete health care. Although men as well as women generally visit more than one doctor as they age, women usually start this fragmented care at adolescence and continue throughout their lives. Why does this happen? One reason is that medical science tends to compartmentalize women's health into physical health and reproductive health, thereby necessitating care by a generalist as well as a gynecologist from puberty onward. In many ways, however, the reliance on medical specialties has improved the health of women. For example, women have been the beneficiaries of advancements that have resulted in a 90 percent decline in maternal mortality—from 73.7 deaths for every 100,000 births in 1950 to 7.3 deaths for every 100,000 births in 1989.

Tip

The most important step a woman can take to improve health status is to choose the correct doctor, a primary care doctor, to consolidate and coordinate care. There are three possible choices:

- *Internist*
- *Obstetrician/Gynecologist*
- *Family Practitioner*

While health care reforms are likely to change the trend toward medical specialization, the burden still rests on individual women to structure the kind of comprehensive health care that will serve them properly.

Choosing a Doctor

The most important step a woman can take to improve health status is to choose the correct doctor, a primary care doctor, to consolidate and coordinate care. There are three possible choices:

Internist

For comprehensive care you would do well to choose this specialist, who is trained to treat general medical problems. Some internists subspecialize in fields that especially apply to women (and men) such as cardiovascular disease, endocrinology, and rheumatology. You may want to select an internist if you have a family or personal history of heart disease, gastrointestinal problems, diabetes, or arthritis.

Obstetrician/Gynecologist

Although these specialists are not trained to treat general medical conditions, many women do, indeed, receive excellent care in obstetrician/gynecologists' offices. You may select this specialist if you have a family or personal history of uterine, cervical, or ovarian cancer or if you are concerned about family planning and/or fertility.

Family Practitioner

This specialist receives very broad training that covers internal medicine as well as obstetrics and gynecology.

You may select a family practice specialist if you prefer that every member of your family—including children—receive their health care from one doctor. Family practice is an emerging specialty in medical practice today; however, in many urban medical centers, the family practitioner may not be given broad privileges, such as surgical and obstetrics.

Do Women Need Women Doctors?

It's no secret that women and men are different, but the question is whether women bring to medical work certain characteristics that make for more effective medical care, especially for women patients.

> *According to two recent studies, female doctors do seem to perform certain purely medical functions better than their male counterparts.*

According to two recent studies, female doctors do seem to perform certain purely medical functions better than their male counterparts. A research project published in the *New England Journal of Medicine* showed that female internists and family practitioners were twice as likely to order mammograms and Pap tests as were men in the same specialties. Another study published in the journal *Medical Care* found a similar pattern.

There's more to medical care than ordering tests, however. Evidence suggests that women doctors do in fact, communicate differently with patients than men doctors do. Specifically, they use more positive terms, compliments, and agreements, and they use more partnership statements, which say, in effect,

"We are going to work on this together." Women doctors also encourage more talk from patients, which not only generates a sense of trust but also brings to light certain emotional problems that may affect health. These factors include how you experience your illness, how you are coping with it, and what elements of treatment are important to you.

Women doctors also tend to spend more time with patients. After analyzing 500 audiotaped office visits, researchers at the Johns Hopkins University School of Hygiene and Public Health in Baltimore found, in general, that female doctors tend to ask a lot more questions about medical history, pay far more attention to patients' feelings, and that, from start to finish, patients (and that includes male patients, too) spent more time face-to-face with female doctors than with male doctors.

In the final analysis, finding a female doctor is not as important as finding a doctor who, besides being well trained and competent, is sensitive to your needs as a patient.

The Basic Exams

There are no set rules for what makes up an annual checkup. Therefore, you should have a clear idea of what services you want performed when you visit your primary care doctor for a general health evaluation. These components could be included in your annual physical exam, depending on your age, prior health status, and the degree of risk the test may pose to you.

The Medical Evaluation

- Complete medical history—to allow your doctor to consider your present medical status in context with past medical history and assessments.
- Comprehensive physical—a careful analysis of your body from hair and eyes to ankles and toes to detect medical abnormalities.
- Urine and stool samples—analysis of color, amount, and contents to detect potential diseases.
- Chest X-ray—to assess lungs, heart, major blood vessels in the chest, and the bony cage that houses the thoracic contents. Women who smoke or who are at risk for tuberculosis should make a point of discussing this test with their doctors.
- Electrocardiogram—an indirect depiction of the heart's electrical activity to detect disturbances in heart rhythm. Women with a family history of certain types of heart disease should have this test periodically.
- Blood pressure measurements—to determine pressure of your blood's flow against the walls of the arteries and detect possible elevated readings.
- Sigmoidoscopy—a complete direct look at the lower portion of the intestinal tract—anus, rectum, and sigmoid—to detect polyps, hemorrhoids, or cancer. The test is generally not appropriate for women under the age of 35 who do not have a family history of colorectal cancer.
- Blood tests—a complete blood count (CBC) to provide information on red and white blood cells, as well as data on sugar content, uric acid, potassi-

um, calcium, phosphorus, cholesterol, and several enzymes that reveal status of kidneys, liver, and other internal organs, including abnormalities of blood.

The Gynecologic Evaluation

- Complete obstetric and gynecologic history—to allow your doctor to consider your present gynecologic status in context with past gynecologic assessments.
- Menstrual history assessment—to determine possible causes of premenstrual problems and institute preventive treatment.
- Pelvic exam—to detect anatomical or structural abnormalities as well as any discharges or suspicious growths.
- Pap test—to detect cancer of the uterus at the very earliest stages before a tumor actually develops.
- Breast examination—to ensure early detection of cancerous growths and commence preventive treatment for chronic cysts.
- Mammogram—to detect breast lumps that are too small to be felt during regular breast examination. Recommended at various ages depending on family history.
- Bladder function assessment—to assess possible causes of incontinence.
- Contraceptive evaluation—to determine if current contraceptive practices are effective and appropriate.

Different Health Concerns across Your Life Span

Different conditions affect women at different times in their lives. In general:

Younger women are concerned with illnesses and conditions that, while they are not life threatening, often necessitate frequent contact with health care providers. These include gynecological infections, sexually transmitted diseases, emotional disorders, autoimmune diseases, and eating disorders. Many younger women are also concerned with all aspects of reproduction from family planning to fertility.

Older women are primarily concerned with chronic conditions associated with aging and changes in hormones. In some respects, the conditions of concern become more similar to the concerns of their male counterparts: heart disease, lung cancer, cerebrovascular disease, and diabetes in addition to cervical cancer, ovarian cancer, breast cancer, osteoporosis, and Alzheimer's disease.

For women in metropolitan areas, the search for a primary care doctor specializing in the concerns of younger or older women is fairly easy. Most large hospital centers actually promote this kind of specialized care in the form of free informative brochures or open lectures to which the public is invited. In a smaller community setting you can still track down doctors with special interests. The director of medicine or director of outpatient services at your nearest hospital should be able to provide you with relevant information.

How to Avoid Overtreatment

Some experts claim that women seek medical care too often. In addition to being the family "gatekeeper," controlling and directing the family's use of health care, women also read consumer publications that discuss various diseases and medical conditions and respond more actively than men do.

Today, because of advances in diagnostic technology, doctors are able to find more problems than they know how to treat. For example, human papillomavirus (HPV) can be detected very early with a newly developed, highly sensitive test. However, there are no treatments for HPV and certainly no cure. While regular Pap tests that might show changes possibly caused by HPV infection are indicated, some surgeons take an aggressive approach, performing laser surgery that involves considerable pain and even damage to the woman's genitals. Similar cases in point are the overuse of hysterectomies, dilatation of the cervix and curettage of the uterus (D & C), and cesarean sections, all of which are performed far too extensively, say critics.

Tip

There is a saying in the medical profession that goes like this: "If you have a stomachache in France, you get a suppository, in Germany, you go to a health spa, in America, you have an operation."

Part of the reason for overtreatment is that our medical system was designed primarily to cure the sick. There is a saying in the medical profession that goes like this: "If you have a stomachache in France, you get a suppository, in Germany, you go to a health spa, in America, you have an operation." Currently, there is a significant lack of emphasis on the training—and compensation—of doctors for preventive care. But that may soon change, as the health care financing system, emphasis on outcomes, and, ultimately, medical decision-making undergo reform.

Two factors may sway your decision in selecting a hospital: one, whether the hospital includes the services of a specialized center for women's health and, two, whether the hospital offers unique benefits to women preparing for childbirth.

An important protective tool against overtreatment is information. To the best of your ability you should stay well informed.

Choosing a Hospital

Except in the case of emergencies, which may necessitate a trip to the nearest medical facility, most people go to the hospital of their doctor's choice—the place where the primary care doctor has admitting privileges. If a doctor recommends hospitalization, don't hesitate to ask if the hospital is experienced in your type of case. If you are not satisfied that it is, ask to be referred to a hospital in which you would have more confidence. Section Two of this book provides a step-by-step process that will lead you to the best hospital for your particular needs.

Two factors may sway your decision: one, whether the hospital includes the services of a specialized center for women's health and, two, whether the hospital offers unique benefits to women preparing for childbirth.

Women's Health Centers

As the country's current health care system begins to recognize the unique needs of women, hospitals and medical centers are introducing special facilities to provide for those needs. At almost every major medical center in the country, a special women's health center has been, or is about to be, introduced. While these women's health centers are, in part, promotional efforts on the part of the institution, they can, in fact, offer real benefits to women.

Some centers offer targeted care—they are disease-, organ-, or condition-oriented—while others provide comprehensive care. Women's centers specializing in breast care, for example, will offer low-cost mammograms as well as educational material on breast self-examination. Women's centers targeted to women who are approaching or going through menopause focus diagnostic and treatment options on the physical and psychological problems that women encounter during the 30 or so years that make up the climacteric or pre- through post-menopause period.

Tip

Hospital-based centers for women's health focus on optimizing health and well-being through fitness evaluations and preventive health care.

Comprehensive centers for women's health, on the other hand, address a broad range of health concerns.

The doctors associated with these centers represent a range of specialties, such as cardiology, dermatology, endocrinology, general internal medicine, gynecology, obstetrics, nutrition, preventive medicine, psychiatry, rehabilitation medicine, reproductive medicine, surgery, urology, and other key areas. These centers for women's health focus on optimizing health and well-being through fitness evaluations and preventive health care. Moreover, the centers usually provide an environment conducive to attracting a population of healthy working women, most of whom would prefer to avoid a hospital setting. The most attractive aspect for such women is easy access to services and rapid test results all available in one place.

▼

A buyer in a large department store in San Francisco is typical of the busy women who support these new centers for women's health. Before the introduction of the center in a hospital near her workplace two years ago, she had let three years pass since her last Pap test and, at the age of 45, had never had a mammogram. Now, the tests are part of the annual examination that she can schedule at her convenience without sacrificing additional time for separate appointments.

▼

Childbirth facilities

In the case of childbirth there is usually an ample nine months in which to choose a hospital and that choice is usually made when you select an obstetrician because these specialists typically limit their deliveries to one or, at most, two hospitals. The two factors that can determine the most appropriate choice are prenatal care and personal needs.

Prenatal care. The vast majority of deliveries are uncomplicated. Deliveries that might require specialized hospital services can be identified well in advance of birth during prenatal examinations by the doctor. Prospective parents should discuss the labor and delivery procedures with the obstetrician. One important piece of information to be learned is the hospital's cesarean section rate. Preferably, the figure should be 30 percent or less and higher numbers should be questioned unless the hospital specializes in high-risk obstetrics. While a C-section is strongly recommended for a second delivery in certain situations (such as when the mother has genital herpes), the procedure should not be used simply because you had one previously.

Tip

Choose a hospital with a C-section rate of 30 percent or less.

The American College of Obstetricians and Gynecologists (ACOG) has confirmed the safety and advisability of vaginal birth after a cesarean (VBAC) for the vast majority of women. However ACOG recommends that hospitals offering VBAC be prepared to start emergency cesarean surgery and anesthesia within 30 minutes of the time the decision is made. As precautions, continuous fetal monitoring and 24–hour access to blood bank facilities are advised.

Personal needs. Many hospitals, prompted by forward-thinking obstetricians, offer a delivery room that resembles a home environment and encourages family members to attend the delivery. You may want to find out if the hospital has nurse midwives on staff; the presence of these professionals indicates a hospital's commitment to a variety of birthing options. Many hospitals offer a range of childbirth education classes and support groups for interested parents. Even for parents-to-be who are not sold on the idea of natural childbirth techniques, the programs can provide valuable information on the care and feeding of infants and children.

Tip

When choosing an HMO, you should look for a variety of screening programs as well as periodic medical examinations.

As for the basics, you should check out the obstetrical service of the hospitals under consideration. Talk to your doctor, friends, and the appropriate hospital spokesperson—in this case the administrator or director of obstetrical nursing—to assess the labor room procedures. In the end, the decision may rest on the number of babies that enter the world each day in a given hospital; the more babies delivered, the better equipped and staffed the hospital probably is to handle the broadest range of obstetrical needs. If there is any possibility of a problem during childbirth, you should be sure that the hospital has a neonatal or pediatric intensive care unit.

A final word: when you are investigating various hospital services, be sure that the hospital has a mammography program certified by the American College of Radiology or the Food and Drug Administration (see Appendix N).

Choosing an HMO

Since the cornerstone of managed care is prevention of illness and disability, a major factor in considering one managed care program over another is its emphasis on comprehensive care of women.

You should look for a variety of screening programs as well as periodic medical examinations. The specific coverages to investigate include physical exams, prenatal and postnatal care, family planning, well-baby care, and laboratory diagnostic tests. Most important is whether the HMO not only lists these services but makes sure that they are frequently used. Some HMO report cards give data on the use of these services by members. In addition, consider the number of wellness programs or health promotion initiatives offered by the managed care program. These include programs for stopping smoking, weight control, stress management, and breast self-examination. An outstanding HMO offers a selection of classes, courses, newsletters, and resource guides for members.

Even with serious and chronic conditions such as diabetes, arthritis, chronic pulmonary disorders, and heart failure, there is strong evidence that complications can be avoided and the need for medical services reduced through effective day-to-day management by the patient under the overall direction of the primary care doctor. The best managed care program is the one that offers provisions for such management.

Procedures and Products to Question

Medical science seems to be moving away from the notion that women's natural biological processes are treatable illnesses. As it does, women will no longer be subjected to the commercialization of treatment for normal female functions, such as menstruation, lactation, and menopause. But until the trend is reversed, you need to examine with a critical eye those treatments and techniques that may be overused. These include:

- Estrogen replacement therapy. There is a great deal of controversy over this subject, which is also called hormone replacement therapy (HRT). More than three and one half million women begin estrogen replacement therapy in a given year to alleviate menopausal symptoms such as hot flashes, vaginal dryness, and mood changes, as well as to lower their risk of heart disease. However, there is a lack of conclusive evidence that this hormone, when taken in combination with a synthetic form of the naturally occurring hormone progesterone, will lower the rate at which women die of heart disease. In addition, many women take estrogen replacement therapy to prevent osteoporosis although they are at little or no risk of developing the disease.
- Cesarean section. At the current rate, one in four women in the United States will deliver a baby by cesarean section. Consumer interest groups estimate that 50 percent of the cesare-

an sections performed in this country are unnecessary. However, there is a growing awareness in the medical profession of this situation, and efforts are being made to reduce the number of C-sections.

- Hysterectomy. At the current rate, one in three women in the United States will have a hysterectomy before reaching the age of 60. According to estimates of consumer interest groups, approximately one quarter of all hysterectomies performed in a given year (about 150,000) are unnecessary.

- Weight loss products. More than 20 million people a year—mostly women—use diet-aid products, spending more than $300 million a year. While this category includes special food products, which are not harmful, per se, the bulk of the products are in the form of medications whose active ingredient is similar to amphetamines or drugs that are used as "speed" or "uppers."

- Breast implants. More than two million women have breast implants either for cosmetic augmentation or reconstruction following mastectomy. Silicone gel breast implants have been implicated in numerous complications, including allergic and autoimmune reactions, infections, and implant failures. Saline breast implants have also come under scrutiny.

Assessing the use of these products and procedures judiciously may not only save you money but also improve your health.

A Changing Research Perspective

The 16th-century French essayist, Montaigne, wrote: "Women are not entirely wrong when they reject the rules of life prescribed for the world, for they were established by men only, without their consent." Montaigne might have written the same words in this century—indeed until the last decade—especially with regard to the rules of medical care that have been forged from a reliance on the male model of what is medically normal for a human being.

In 1990, that began to change. Bernadine Healy, MD, upon assuming her position as the first woman director of the National Institutes of Health (NIH), created the Office of Research on Women's Health (ORWH) to make sure that women and women's health issues were included in all NIH-funded studies. And further, to correct the research imbalance, Dr. Healy announced the Women's Health Initiative (WHI), a $625 million, 14-year project that began in the autumn of 1993. The initiative is designed to examine the major causes of death, disease, and frailty in more than 140,000 older women of all races and socioeconomic backgrounds. It is the largest health study ever done at the NIH.

The Women's Health Initiative (WHI), a $625 million, 14-year project of the National Institutes of Health, will examine the major causes of death, disease, and frailty in more than 140,000 older women of all races and socioeconomic backgrounds. It is the largest health study ever done at the NIH.

Recently, this country has witnessed higher appropriations for research on ovarian cancer to $26.2 million, nearly five times the amount spent in 1988. Meanwhile, the Food and Drug Administration's (FDA) drug approval process was called into question by the federal government's General Accounting Office; it was found that women are often underrepresented in FDA studies and have not been analyzed separately from men.

In 1991 the Pharmaceutical Manufacturers Association, a Washington-based industry trade association, announced the results of a survey that indicated that the industry is now testing 263 new medications for use by women.

These efforts, and others, will hopefully make up ground for women who, as Emily Friedman describes in the United Hospital Fund of New York's new book, *An Unfinished Revolution: Women and Health Care in America,* "have often been at a disadvantage in terms of the resources and autonomy allowed them by the health care system; they have been disproportionately victimized by unnecessary care, as well as dismissal of symptoms as nothing more than emotional turmoil or menses."

The health status of American women is at a crossroads. In order to move in a forward direction toward superior health outcomes and quality of life, the factors that reflect gaps in knowledge about how to prevent and treat illnesses in women must be addressed. While changes in the health care system and improved research can close some of the gaps, it is up to individual women to optimize their own health care and thereby maximize their productivity and enjoyment of life.

The Special Health Care Needs of Children

Chapter 25

Although childhood is often viewed as a carefree, blissful time, the fact of the matter is that children get sick—and they do so with great regularity. While the scourges of the past—polio, smallpox, measles, and diphtheria—have been largely conquered by remarkable medical advances, parents today still have a host of concerns ranging from nuisance conditions such as the common cold to potential environmental hazards in the form of pesticides and pollution.

Further, according to the National Center for Health Statistics, children under the age of 18 suffer from many of the same chronic illnesses that plague adults:

- Hay fever and respiratory allergies afflict more than five and one-half million children.
- Ear infections strike about five and three-quarter million children each year.
- Asthma is experienced by nearly two and one-quarter million children.
- Severe headaches strike nearly two million children.
- Digestive disorders affect about one-half million children.

Keeping children healthy has never been an easy job. As principal guardians of a child's healthy growth and development, parents need a unique combination of experience and knowledge in order to maintain a child's good health. From these two sources come the confidence to make wise health care choices.

A new subspecialty, adolescent medicine, has recently been recognized by the American Board of Pediatrics and the American Board of Internal Medicine.

Choosing a Doctor

A child's doctor has a unique and intimate relationship with parents as well as patient. You should approach the process of choosing the proper doctor with great care from the start, in order to avoid making disruptive changes in health care providers. There are two possible choices:

Pediatrician

This specialist is trained in the care of children from infancy through adolescence. You should look for a board-certified pediatrician (don't assume, ask for credentials), and an assurance that the doctor is prepared to treat all general medical conditions of childhood. Some pediatricians are also board-certified in a subspecialty, such as cardiology, endocrinology, gastroenterology, or infectious diseases. In addition, a new subspecialty, adolescent medicine, has recently been recognized by the American Board of Pediatrics and the American Board of Internal Medicine.

Family Practitioner

This specialist has very broad training in disciplines that cover adult care as well as children's health care. While most children begin their health care in a pediatrician's office, a family practitioner may also assume care of children from infancy. A family practitioner may be an appropriate choice if you want your family's health care to come from a single source. Family practice is an emerging specialty in medical practice today; however, in many urban medical centers, the family practitioner may not be given broad privileges and, in some cases, may not be granted admitting privileges at certain hospitals.

A Pediatrician's Role

So-called baby doctors often say that they are part physician, part psychologist, and part philosopher, since, in addition to providing medical treatment, much of their time is spent in answering parents' questions and allaying fears. Here is a job description for a good pediatrician:

- Offers prenatal advice about nutrition, medication, and parental attitudes toward the baby.
- Conducts a newborn physical exam and gives information and advice on feeding and early infant care.
- Conducts well-baby examinations to follow growth and development, administers immunizations, provides advice on feeding and exercise.
- Diagnoses and treats minor illnesses or injuries with medical advice and/or drugs.
- Diagnoses and treats emergencies and serious illnesses with highly technical knowledge,

equipment, and medications.

- Provides advice and answers to questions by telephone at designated times.
- Refers unique and complicated problems to appropriate subspecialists.

Getting the Most from Your Child's Doctor

Many parents feel that they have little or no influence over what happens to their child or to them in a doctor's office. Actually, parents do have significant control. The more actively you participate in your child's health care, the more likely you are to get what you want. Here are some suggestions that can help you develop a strong partnership with the doctor of your choice:

- Make a list of questions before each appointment and make sure all questions are answered to your satisfaction before the appointment is over.
- Express any disagreement you feel about a treatment plan immediately and frankly so it can be resolved.
- Make the doctor aware of possible problems in following a prescribed treatment.
- Telephone the doctor if unexpected problems arise, if worries persist, or if the treatment doesn't seem to be working.
- Make the doctor aware of financial problems at the onset so that the most economical treatment regi-

mens can be prescribed and appropriate payment methods set up.

- Determine who will cover for the doctor, if necessary.

The Well-Baby Exam

A physical examination consists of experienced general observation of a child and consideration of specific symptoms. The office visit is not a mysterious ritual; each step is designed to elicit specific information.

Here is what makes up a typical physical exam:

- History—to allow the doctor to consider the child's health status in the context of pregnancy and delivery problems and the family health history.
- Weight and height measurements—to give an indication of the child's growth pattern over time and in relation to normal growth curves.
- General appearance—to assess a child's look of health relative to normal/abnormal appearances of other children.
- Specific examination of skin, limbs, face, eyes, ears, head, neck, mouth, throat, chest, heart, abdomen, genitalia, anus—to establish a record that will serve as a context against which future evaluations are compared as well as to detect any defects and abnormalities.
- Motor and neurological function—to evaluate the normal functioning of muscles and the central and peripheral nervous systems as well as to assess developmental status.

Your Child and the Doctor

In the first few months of life, most infants are quite comfortable with visits to the doctor. While the coldness of instruments, sharpness of needles for injections, or being forced to stretch and turn may bring on cries of complaint, a child's memory is short-lived when it comes to such discomfort.

Tip

Because of early negative experiences in a doctor's office, many children grow up with a strong fear and dislike for a major source of good health in their lives.

Between six months and three years of age, the dynamic changes. For one thing, most children develop classic separation anxiety at this time and also begin to feel uncomfortable around strangers. Moreover, babies will develop conditioned responses to unpleasant experiences—injections and unfamiliar instruments, in particular.

By the age of three, children begin to develop fears and phobias about sickness and death. In most cases, the doctor becomes a stranger who is inflicting unwanted handling and even discomfort and pain.

Little wonder, then, that many children grow up with a strong fear and dislike for a major source of good health in their lives. There is recourse, however. If parents simply realize that a child may be upset by a visit to the doctor, they can handle the situation in a more reasonable way, thereby making it easier for the child:

One: Be frank and open about the doctor and educate children about the doctor, the office, and the tools. For example, it is unwise to tell a child that an injection "won't hurt a bit," when, in fact, it will probably hurt a lot, although only for a minute.

Two: Provide a safety zone for children during the office visit by remaining close by, holding them during the exam, and providing favorite toys and security items.

Three: Never, under any circumstance, threaten to punish a child who is misbehaving with a "trip to the doctor."

Four: Don't show signs of your own fears and anxieties in front of your child.

Choosing a Hospital

In general, children's hospitals provide the best, most specialized, and most complete care for their small patients. There are 131 hospitals in the United States devoted solely to the care of children, ranging from infancy through adolescence. These hospitals provide routine treatment as well as highly specialized and innovative care for complicated problems.

Some of these children's hospitals specialize in life-threatening diseases, while others focus on particular problems, such as orthopedic cases, that may require long-term rehabilitation. All children's hospitals are staffed by a multidisciplinary team of pediatric specialists and subspecialists, as well as nurses, social workers, play therapists, and other support personnel who are trained to work with children. In addition to treating very complex medical problems, children's hospitals are also especially prepared to meet the emotional needs of young patients and their families.

However, since these hospitals are generally found only in large metropolitan areas, they are not easily accessible for families who live in smaller cities and towns. Most parents, therefore, will rely on well-developed pediatric units at local community hospitals and academic medical centers. These specialized units are staffed by pediatricians with one or more subspecialties, highly trained pediatric nurses, and a full complement of pediatric equipment.

Even in communities too small to offer a specialized unit for children's care, some routine procedures—tonsillectomy, setting broken bones, appendectomy, for example—can still be performed in the local hospital, providing the anesthesiology department has appropriate pediatric equipment and doctors on staff. Although there is no board-certified subspecialty in pediatric anesthesia, you should make certain that the anesthesia is administered by someone with training in children, especially in major

The Routine Exam: How Often?

Assuming that a child is basically healthy, the physical exams should take place:

- *Up to age one—every one to two months.*
- *Age one to age two—three or four times a year.*
- *Age two to age six—twice a year.*
- *Age six and above—once a year.*
- *Adolescents—once a year, because of the variety of developmental and related sexual problems that can occur during this span of years.*

surgery. Your pediatrician or family care practitioner should know about the expertise of the hospital to which he or she has admitting privileges.

The distinct advantage of a local hospital in the case of hospitalized children is closeness to home, which allows for parental visits and support. While family support is important to all patients, it is vital in the care and recovery of children. In fact, many hospitals offer special accommodations for a parent who wants to stay close by a child immediately following admission and/or surgery. If you want to stay with your child and the hospital discourages it, you should take an assertive stance. You can ask your doctor to write an "order" or you can argue that you have a legal right to remain since you are the one giving consent for treatment.

Several years ago, in a large Brooklyn, New York, hospital, young patients spoke of their apprehensions to a staff member who recorded them in a booklet. Here are some of them: "This doll needs hundreds of shots because he's been bad, very bad. He hit his sister and then he came into the hospital." "The needle feels like a cold, sharp icicle pushing into my arm. The doctor is trying to push it all the way to my brain." "I know what is happening to all the blood they are taking from my arm. The nurses hide it in dark closets and then the doctors come along and drink it." These revelations illustrate how terrifying hospitalization can be for a child; one study found that during the first 24 hours of hospitalization, a child is exposed to an average of 54 contacts with different people, many of them associated with pain or frightening equipment. Many hospitals do a very good job of advance preparation, such as holding a "pre-op party" before the actual hospital admission where children are shown stuffed animals wearing hospital gowns, stretchers, wagons, breathing masks, stethoscopes, and other equipment that will be used during the hospital stay. If the hospital your child is going to does not have these programs, you should try some preparation yourself. For useful advice on how to help children get ready for hospitalization, contact Children in Hospitals now the Association for the Care of Children's Health (see Appendix L). Or visit your local library which may have a selection of books dealing with this topic.

Tip

Many hospitals arrange with the public school system to provide visiting teachers, an important plus for school-age children who can maintain their schoolwork and, thereby, avoid being left behind their schoolmates.

If the hospital stay is going to be lengthy, you should investigate the quality-of-life services that will be provided to your child. A child life program can provide enormous benefits in terms of psychological healing. Such programs, usually with a playroom as the nucleus, offer an opportunity to experience some of the patterns of everyday living activities in a housekeeping corner, for example, designed to reproduce the basics of home. Many hospitals arrange with the public school system to provide visiting teachers, an important plus for school age children who can maintain their schoolwork and, thereby, avoid being left behind their schoolmates.

For conditions of a complicated or serious nature—for example, open-heart surgery, neurological evaluations, severe head injuries, or exploratory abdominal surgery—you will want the most up-to-date and sophisticated medical or surgical care available. If your local hospital does not offer the range of services your child may need, seek out the services at a larger academic medical center or specialized children's hospital.

Choosing an HMO

In choosing an HMO for your family, you should consider how strong an emphasis the plan places on the health care of children.

Tip

In choosing an HMO for your family, you should consider how strong an emphasis the plan places on the health care of children in its range of coverages.

You should look for a variety of screening programs as well as periodic medical examinations. The specific coverages to investigate include physical exams, well-baby care, and laboratory diagnostic tests. Make sure all immunizations are covered. In addition, find out if the hospitals used by the HMO have good pediatric units as well as an adequate number of well-trained pediatricians and pediatric subspecialists available.

HMOs also offer wellness programs for patients, special programs on nutrition and fitness for children, and educational materials for parents on these and other relevant subjects. These special services should be considered in making a choice of a plan.

Tip

If there is a single important step you can take toward ensuring continued good health care for your child, it is creating a complete and documented medical history and personal health record.

Your Child's Medical History

To new parents, a baby's weight gains and walking progress are of great emotional value. But they have important medical implications, as well. All medical facts provide a background against which to measure present health status. Just possibly, a long forgotten fact of a childhood disease can provide an important clue to a medical mystery some years hence. If there is a single important step you can take toward ensuring continued good health care for your child, it is creating a complete and documented medical history and personal health record. This record follows an individual throughout life and the earlier it is begun, the better it will aid health care providers.

A medical history is a résumé of everything medically significant throughout your child's life, including facts about health as well as details of illnesses. Among the many items contained in your child's medical history should be:

- Vital signs—normal body temperature, pulse rate, respiratory rate, blood pressure.
- Growth statistics—weight, height, other important measurements.
- Developmental records—rate of progress in

acquiring new skills.

- Immunization records.
- Childhood diseases—chicken pox, repeated infections, measles, German measles, mumps, whooping cough, etc. (If your child is fully immunized, he/she is unlikely to contract these.)
- Allergies/asthma record.
- Chronic illness record.
- Medication records.
- Corrective devices.
- Accidents, injuries.
- Surgical record.
- Family history.

A final word of advice: While you should always press for the best medical care, some parents have a tendency to overreact to normal childhood problems, making unreasonable demands on the child's doctor.

One example of this is the case of the mother who brought her child to a pediatrician to be examined for hearing loss. Upon examination, the doctor found that the child had an ear infection which involved considerable fluid accumulation around the ear drum. When she advised the mother of the real problem, noting that the fluid was impeding the child's hearing, and that it would be senseless to conduct a hearing test under such conditions, the mother was still insistent on testing.

▼

The Special Health Care Needs of Older Adults

Chapter 26

While this chapter addresses health care and related concerns of older Americans in their post-retirement years, it is also intended for those who will be the primary caregivers of the elderly.

If you are one of the millions of Americans who is or soon will be over 65, it's never too early to plan for the special health care needs that often accompany the aging process. This is also true if you have a parent or other relative who is in this group, because caring for the elderly, or "elder care," is expected to take up more resources in the coming decades than child care. Statistics show that by 2005, 37 percent of US workers will be aged 40 to 54, the prime time for caring for elderly parents. And, according to the Census Bureau, the number of people 85 and older who rely on their children will nearly double by 2030 and more than triple by 2050, with families providing 80 percent of needed long-term care.

Most of us look forward to our later years as a time to be free from the stresses and demands of careers and raising families, while pursuing our own interests. What we often don't envision, however, are the potential health care concerns, and accompanying lifestyle changes, that may derail our plans for the future. While body parts don't all age at the same rate, at around age 30 our immune systems begin to decline in effectiveness, making us increasingly vulnerable to everything from the common cold to cancer. So, in general, the older we are, the less able our bodies are to fight disease.

Average life expectancy in 1900 was only 47 years. Today it is 76 years. The fastest-growing age group of our population is that over 85. The fact that so many of us will be living longer than our forebears introduces a whole new set of health care concerns hardly witnessed in previous centuries. Arthritis, cancer, heart disease, and dementia were as rare in the last century as a 60th birthday. Even the loss of physical strength or the inability to keep up with everyday chores such as cleaning, shopping, and cooking can hinder a healthy or independent existence.

According to the Census Bureau, the number of people 85 and older who rely on their children will nearly double by 2030 and more than triple by 2050, with families providing 80 percent of needed long-term care.

While aging doesn't have to mean illness or a restricted lifestyle, there are, obviously, problems associated with getting older that can be, if not prevented, at least prepared for when they are anticipated. Choosing the right doctor, health care coverage, and lifestyle option before you are confronted with any of these problems can help to make those later years healthier and happier.

Choosing a Doctor

Just as medicine has greatly changed over the last century, so has the doctor-patient relationship. The Norman Rockwell version of the family doctor who made house calls and treated generations of the same family has fallen by the wayside. Many people now have more impersonal relationships with their doctors or don't routinely go to any doctor. Doctors may retire or die, leaving many patients reluctant to find new doctors. For the elderly, in particular, this practice can be problematic. If you are in such a situation and avoid seeking a source of preventive care, you may end up in the care of a specialist who isn't experienced in managing older patients with complicating health risks.

Tip

Because of the special medical problems associated with aging, it is important for the older patient to find a doctor who has a specific interest in caring for the elderly, if at all possible.

Because of the special medical problems associated with aging, it is important for the older patient to find a doctor who has a specific interest in caring for the elderly, if at all possible. It would be nice if all older patients could have access to doctors with training in geriatrics. However, since these specialists are in short supply, a primary care doctor who is interested in caring for the elderly is the next best thing.

When selecting a doctor, it is imperative to choose a skilled professional who is board-certified, has a good reputation among peers, office staff, and patients, and whose office and practice arrangements suit your needs; for instance, by providing coverage and phone consultations by other doctors during vacations and days off. Once you've identified such a candidate, the next step is to set up an interview to assess your level of comfort with the doctor on both professional and personal levels. Here are 10 questions that can help you reach a decision.

Ten Questions to Help You Choose a Doctor

- Does the doctor have a lot of elderly patients?
- Do you and the doctor agree on medical, moral, and ethical issues?
- Are you comfortable with the doctor's appearance, manners, and way of speaking?
- Does the doctor understand your religious and cultural background (if that is important to you)?
- Are you comfortable talking to the doctor about embarrassing topics?
- Do you get the feeling that the doctor is comfortable in your presence?
- Is the doctor open to dealing with certain conditions without medication, if such options are available?
- Does the doctor emphasize preventive measures for the elderly?
- Will the doctor coordinate your medical care with other specialists, if necessary?
- Does the doctor accept—even encourage—your wish to have a family member or friend accompany you to the doctor's office?

Choosing a Hospital

Most people don't think about choosing a hospital until a medical crisis has occurred and then they usually let their doctor select one for them. But like every other aspect of health care, the elderly consumer should be more proactive when it comes to hospitalization. Not all hospitals are the same, especially in terms of reputation, resources, and services. Some community hospitals, while small and not specialized, may provide high-quality nursing care while some larger medical centers may provide higher-tech facilities with less personalized care. Of course, the selection of a hospital may be based upon the nature of the medical problem (for instance, not all hospitals may provide dialysis for kidney problems). Knowing the hospitals in your area and being able to discuss the options knowledgeably with your doctor is one more step in maintaining control over your health care.

Tip

Knowing the hospitals in your area and being able to discuss the options knowledgeably with your doctor is one more step in maintaining control over your health care.

As with choosing a doctor, you would do well to find a hospital that specializes in the problems of the older patient. However, although there are hospitals that have units devoted to geriatric care, they are few and far between. One indication that a hospital has some interest in elder care is an affiliated nursing home, hospice, or home care program. Being cared for by a doctor who is on the staff of such a hospital may be important if you find yourself or a family member needing care over a long period of time. If the hospital has both acute-care and long-term care capabilities, it may mean a way to avoid a change of hospitals or doctors. The kind of information you need to evaluate the hospitals in your area is outlined in Section Two of this book. Most of the information can be obtained from the hospital's public relations or community relations offices or from an annual report. You can also call your state department of health for information.

Choosing Health Care Coverage That Pays

Your main objective is to choose coverage that will protect both your health and your pocketbook. Here is a review of what is available:

Medicare/Medigap

Health care reform notwithstanding, most older Americans rely and will continue to rely on Medicare to provide the medical insurance coverage they require. In general, beneficiaries are required to pay 20 percent of covered medical services as well as hospital deductibles, co-payments, and the cost of prescription drugs. For those who are relatively healthy, this coverage may be sufficient. But for people with serious or chronic illnesses, the costs incurred by the individual or family can wipe out a life's savings rather quickly.

To address these lapses in coverage, private insurance to supplement Medicare is available. Known as

Medigap policies, the regulations that governed these plans were overhauled by Congress in 1990, resulting in legislation mandating the creation of 10 standardized Medigap policies, lettered A (the basic package) through J. Insurers in all states are required to offer plan A, but may offer the others at their discretion. All of the plans include the core benefits offered in plan A. Not all policies may be available in all states, and prices may vary from insurer to insurer. But each individual plan is identical from insurer to insurer, regardless of cost. So it pays to shop around. To find out which plans are available in your state, call your state insurance department (see Appendix H).

Medigap policies are private insurance policies designed to supplement Medicare.

Obviously, the more coverage you want, the more it is going to cost. Depending on where you live, the basic plan, A, may cost as little as $300 to $400 a year and plan J, the most comprehensive, can cost as much as $2,000 a year. To find out which plans are available in your state, contact your state insurance department. Then seek out the companies that offer the plan of your choice. (For more about each plan, see Appendix J.)

Keep in mind that insurers are prohibited from checking on the health of new applicants age 65 and older for six months after they sign up for Medicare Part B (medical services). So if you have any type of chronic illness, it's important to buy a Medicare supplement policy before the six months are up. Otherwise, you may find it difficult and expensive to obtain any insurance coverage. If you're already covered under a Medigap policy and are satisfied with your coverage, you don't have to switch to a new plan, particularly if your current policy pays for such amenities as private duty nurses. The new plans no longer provide coverage for these services.

Choosing an HMO

Many Health Maintenance Organizations (HMOs) can serve to fill in the gaps of Medicare coverage. Whether or not these HMOs are better or worse than Medigap policies depends upon your needs and the HMO. HMOs' advantages are that they can be less expensive than conventional insurance plans, they may provide all your medical care in one place, and they may offer more services than those traditionally covered under Medicare. On the other hand, some recipients don't like having their choice of doctors and facilities restricted. Also, HMOs are not yet policed as rigidly as traditional insurance providers. As a result, some HMOs can make receiving certain costly benefits, such as skilled nursing or home care, difficult for the elderly. According to an article in *Consumer Reports,* some HMOs have been known to drag out the process of paying for these benefits so long that Medicare beneficiaries have died before ever receiving care they were legally entitled to! The trick is to choose a high-quality HMO!

Tip

Insurers are prohibited from checking on the health of new applicants age 65 and older for six months after they sign up for Medicare Part B (medical services).

HMOs that contract with Medicare to provide services to beneficiaries use one of three methods, which affect how members obtain medical services and what they pay for them. In the first method, known as risk contracts, Medicare pays the HMO a monthly sum to provide all the coverage for beneficiaries who join. The HMO is obligated to provide all Part A (hospital) and Part B (medical) services. In turn, the HMO usually charges members a monthly premium to cover the cost of Medicare deductibles and co-payments. HMOs that offer risk contracts must take all applicants regardless of their health, except those with end-stage kidney disease and those already in a Medicare hospice program. Members of risk contract HMOs are locked into using the HMO's services and are therefore not permitted to seek care outside of the network.

HMOs contract with Medicare to provide services to beneficiaries in one of three ways: risk contracts, cost contracts and health care prepayment plans.

In the second type of service provided by HMOs, known as cost contracts, Medicare pays the HMO a fee to provide hospital and medical services. As with risk contracts, the HMO charges monthly premiums that cover Medicare deductibles and co-payments and must accept all older applicants. At the end of the year, if the plan has spent more than Medicare has paid, Medicare reimburses the HMO. Members belonging to an HMO using a cost contract method are not locked into the HMO; that is, they are free to seek medical services outside of the network. Medicare will reimburse them the cost of the care, but the beneficiary will then have to pay the usual co-payments, deductibles, and extra doctors' charges.

Health care prepayment plans, the third contractual method, require that Medicare pay the HMO to provide medical services only, not hospital services. The HMO does not have to cover all medical services but must provide for doctors' visits, X-rays, lab tests, and other diagnostic tests. Beneficiaries can go outside the plan for care, but again are responsible for paying co-payments, deductibles, and extra charges.

What to Look for in an HMO

Since you will receive all your care from the HMO, try to evaluate the plan's services before you sign up. You can ask the following questions of the staff or acquaintances who belong to the same plan.

- How long do you have to wait to get an appointment?
- Are you assigned a doctor who has overall responsibility for your care?
- Can you usually see that doctor when you make an appointment?
- Do doctors take enough time to conduct a thorough examination, provide proper treatment, and explain what is wrong?
- Can you see a specialist if your condition requires it?
- Can you reach the office by telephone to make

an appointment or to ask questions about your treatment and/or continuing problems?

- Is the office staff helpful when you call or when you visit?

Be sure to refer to Section Three of this book for a complete discussion about choosing and using an HMO.

Long-Term Health Care

Because we are living longer, chances are that many of us will find ourselves needing some kind of long-term health care. Currently, about seven million Americans require such care because they are physically or mentally unable to care for themselves, and some 43 percent of Americans currently 65 or older are expected eventually to enter nursing homes. Couple that with the fact that fewer children of aging parents are willing or able to care for them at home, and it becomes very obvious that other options need to be considered. In addition to nursing homes, long-term health care options include home care, adult day-care, hospices, and assisted care.

Nursing Homes

A survey commissioned by the American Association of Homes for the Aging in 1991 found that 60 percent of those surveyed thought that nursing home care was fair to good, while 23 percent considered it poor. Another survey done that year by the Alliance for Aging Research found that the greatest fear among the elderly is not the prospect of being ill or a financial burden but being sent to a home. Nursing homes, whether deservedly or not, have been dogged with the reputation of being prisons where old people go to live out life sentences.

While nursing home scandals have created fear, it is important to realize that there are many excellent nursing homes, and knowing what to look for will help you find one that might be right for your situation. Keep in mind also that nursing homes don't have to be "last stop" solutions. They can also provide care temporarily while an alternative mode of care is lined up.

Typically, nursing homes are grouped into three classes: skilled nursing, intermediate care, and shelter, or custodial, care. Skilled-nursing facilities are usually inhabited by individuals who are unable to care for themselves, are often bedridden, and require around-the-clock care delivered by registered and licensed practical nurses under the direction of a doctor. Intermediate-care homes also provide medical care, but at a level that is less intensive. Usually delivered by nurses and therapists, care in this type of facility aims to rehabilitate the resident to a point where he or she can go home or at least regain or retain as many functions of daily living as possible. Sheltered, or custodial, care facilities provide residents with assistance in routine activities such as getting out of bed, bathing, eating, and walking but do not usually provide supervised medical treatment.

Tip

Keep in mind also that nursing homes don't have to be "last stop" solutions. They can also provide care temporarily while an alternative mode of care is lined up.

To find out more about nursing homes in your area, begin by asking the potential resident's doctor for recommendations, and check to see if there are any homes affiliated with area hospitals. You should also check with your insurance carrier to see what restrictions they may place on your choice of a facility. More information on nursing home care can be obtained by contacting the American Health Care Association, the American Association of Homes for the Aging, or the National Consumers League (see Appendix L).

Nursing homes are grouped into three classes:

- *Skilled nursing*
- *Intermediate care*
- *Shelter, or custodial, care.*

Home Care

While a nursing home may be the solution that initially comes to mind when you or a loved one becomes debilitated, it is far from the only option worth exploring. Home care is gaining in popularity not only among those who use it but also among government, health, and insurance agencies, which see it as a less expensive option to nursing home care. By enlisting an outside agency to help with services ranging from cooking and cleaning to full nursing care at home, this option permits a person who is no longer able to perform all the tasks associated with daily living to remain in familiar surroundings.

Full-service home health agencies offer everything from skilled nursing care to housekeeping and cooking services. You can usually find a multitude of these agencies listed in the yellow pages, and your doctor or local hospital may be able to direct you to some reputable ones as you begin your search. For information on home health services, contact the Foundation for Hospice and Home Care and the National Association for Home Care (see Appendix L).

Keep in mind that your insurance carrier, if it covers home health care, will probably have restrictions on the type of agency you select, such as whether or not it is certified. For more information on certified home care agencies contact the National League for Nursing–Community Health Accreditation Program or the Joint Commission on Accreditation of Healthcare Organizations (see Appendix L).

Up to 96 percent of the people who attended adult day care centers either improved or maintained their level of function in such activities as bathing, dressing, and problem-solving.

Adult Day Care

When an elderly person who lives alone does not need nursing care or home care, but does need companionship and some kind of daily routine, adult day care may be the solution. According to a year-long study by the California Department of Aging, conducted from 1980 to 1981, up to 96 percent of the people who attended adult day care centers either improved or maintained their levels of function in such activities as bathing, dressing, and problem-solving. The ability to perform these simple daily tasks is crucial in determining whether or not individuals can continue to live on their own. Many day-care services provide door-to-door transportation for their enrollees. Day care, which averages around $40 a day, depending on the region and services, is also much less expensive than home care, which can run anywhere from $8 to $50 an hour. Currently, about 3,000 senior day-care centers are in operation, providing such services as meals, exercise classes, crafts, current events classes, and other activities. To find a facility in your area, call your local department on aging, or refer to the *National Directory of Adult Day Care Centers* (see Appendix P).

Hospices

Hospices are for people who are terminally ill, generally with fewer than six months to live. They are intended to allow dying people to spend their remaining time free from the antiseptic surroundings and life-sustaining technology of a hospital. However, hospices do provide basic medical care, counseling, and prescribed pain relievers. Because they provide only basic medical care, hospices are less expensive than hospitals or nursing homes. Hospices may provide services in the patient's home or they may operate a facility where the patient resides. For more information on hospices near you, ask your doctor or local hospital for a referral or contact the Hospice Education Institute and the National Hospice Organization (see Appendix L).

Assisted Care

Also known as adult congregate-living facilities, assisted living combines housing, skilled and intermediate nursing care, and support services in an apartment-like setting. About one million people currently live in assisted-care communities in this country. As residents require nursing care, they transfer to the nursing home section of the community and, once they recover, return to their apartments. The facility covers all costs of hospitalization and basic fees range from $20 to $100 a day, depending on the types of services needed. Assisted-care facilities also often require a substantial, nonrefundable down payment in addition to these fees. For more information on assisted-care communities, contact the American Association of Homes for the Aging or the American Health Care Association (see Appendix L).

Other Options

For people who don't require constant supervision or a lot of nursing care, there are a number of other options to nursing-home care. Home-maker services can help people by preparing meals and doing housework; Meals on Wheels and similar programs deliver hot meals to the person's home daily; home sharing brings together a group of elderly people under one roof, who might otherwise live alone; telephone reassurance is a system for checking on an elderly person who is housebound and isolated; and shopping services ensure that groceries and other necessities are delivered to the housebound person's home. Although not all communities may offer all of these services, you should contact your local, county, or state welfare or human services agencies to learn about what's available in your area.

> *Tip*
>
> *Medicaid, government-sponsored medical care for the poor, currently covers about half of all nursing home stays.*

How to Pay for Health Care

Even with Medicare, Medigap, and/or HMO coverage, many Americans will find themselves falling short when it comes to paying for long-term care. And, with longer life spans and the economic necessity for two-income households, many of today's families are unable to provide the vigilant care necessary for a parent who is no longer self-sufficient. Statistics indicate that 43 percent of Americans who are currently 65 years old will eventually enter a nursing home. Half of those entering a nursing home will stay less than six months but the other half will stay an average of two and one-half years, at a cost of $30,000 to $40,000 per year. By the year 2010, the cost of a year's stay in a nursing home could easily top $83,000. Medicare and Medigap insurance pay for only a small fraction of skilled nursing care costs. They do not cover extended, intermediate, or custodial care on a long-term basis.

Tip

Medicare and Medigap insurance pay for only a small fraction of skilled nursing care costs. They do not cover extended, intermediate, or custodial care on a long-term basis.

So where do you turn when the money runs out? Medicaid, government-sponsored medical care for the poor, currently covers about half of all nursing home stays. To qualify for Medicaid, a patient's assets cannot exceed a maximum amount specified by the state. Once eligible for Medicaid, a nursing home patient with no spouse or dependents must turn over to the nursing facility all of his or her income, including Social Security checks, except for a small personal-needs allowance of $30 to $50 a month. This procedure, known as spend-down, takes from a person's estate the amount needed, after Social Security, pension, and interest payments, to cover the costs of care. Once the person's savings are liquidated, Medicaid steps in to cover the costs.

In the event that the nursing home resident has a spouse living at home, each state determines how much of a couple's assets the spouse can keep, ranging from a minimum of $13,740 to a maximum of $68,700. The applicant's home, household goods, and personal effects are not counted. However, the state can recoup what its Medicaid program has spent after both spouses die.

Long-Term Health Care Insurance

There are two ways to protect your assets from being consumed by Medicaid spend-down: estate planning devices and long-term health care insurance. If you wish to use estate-planning you should enlist the advice of an attorney. The other method to protect your assets, long-term health care insurance, involves three kinds of policies: those that cover only nursing home stays, those that cover only home care, and those that cover both.

Nursing home coverage can include skilled, intermediate, and custodial care. Skilled care is intensive, around-the-clock medical care by trained, licensed personnel. Intermediate care is also provided by trained professionals but is not as intensive. Custodial, or personal, care helps patients with every-

Once eligible for Medicaid, a nursing home patient with no spouse or dependents must turn over to the nursing facility all of his or her income, including Social Security checks, except for a small personal-needs allowance of $30 to $50 a month.

day activities such as eating, bathing, dressing, and getting around.

Home care coverage, as interpreted by most insurance policies, is necessary medical care provided by skilled professionals such as nurses and occupational, speech, or physical therapists. Some policies will include licensed home health aides who provide personal or custodial care in this definition. And still fewer policies pay for homemaker services such as cooking, cleaning, and running errands. Obviously, the more of these services a policy covers, the better.

In addition to nursing home and home care services, typical coverages offered by leading sellers of long-term care insurance include adult day-care coverage; a five-year to unlimited maximum benefit period; Alzheimer's disease coverage; guaranteed renewability of the contract; inflation consideration; waiver of the premium when the policyholder has begun receiving benefits; a 30-day free-look period; $40 to $120-per-day nursing home daily benefit and $20 to $60-per-day home health care daily benefit; and one to 20-day home health care and 90 to 100-day nursing home deductible period.

All policies have restrictions that determine benefit eligibility. Known as "gatekeepers," these restrictions are the most important part of the policy because they determine whether or not benefits are paid. The least restrictive policies—and the ones you should look for—begin benefits when the policyholder's doctor orders the care. More common are policies that require care to be medically necessary. Many patients who enter nursing homes may not be sick or injured but may require custodial care; hence, their stays may not be medically necessary. Other types of gatekeepers require that policyholders be unable to perform a certain number of "activities of daily living" (ADLs) before benefits will be paid. The six standard ADLs are: bathing, dressing, transferring (between bed and chair, etc.), walking, toileting (and associated personal hygiene), and eating. Some companies may include other abilities, such as taking medicine or mental capabilities, among these ADLs.

When looking for long-term health care insurance, make sure that the policy is as unambiguous as possible. The policies that spell out exactly what they mean by "failure to perform an activity" or "medically necessary" are the least likely to hold any surprises in the future. However, if a policy is very clear but also very restrictive, you should look further. A few policies require that policyholders be unable to perform activities of daily living because of illness or injury—a very restrictive gatekeeper.

Tip

When looking for long-term health care insurance, make sure that the policy is as unambiguous as possible.

Another important point to keep in mind when looking for a policy is inflation protection.

If you purchase a policy at age 65, but don't need it until you're 85, chances are the benefits you signed up for 20 years earlier won't be sufficient to cover the costs of the nursing home of the future. In fact, a nursing home that costs $100 a day now could cost $300 a day in 2014. Not all inflation protection provisions are alike, however, and they should be looked at carefully. One method lets policyholders buy additional coverage every few years at the then current price, based on their age at the time. The price of that additional coverage, however, can go up so rapidly it will become virtually unaffordable. A second method of increasing coverage to account for inflation automatically increases the daily benefit by some percentage each year uncompounded. So a typical $80 benefit that increases 5 percent a year will be worth $160 in 20 years. If that benefit had been compounded it would be worth $212. Most companies that offer inflation protection discontinue increases after 10 or 20 years. Only a few companies continue inflation increases for the life of the policy.

Tip

An important point to keep in mind when looking for a policy is inflation protection.

Paying for inflation protection can be expensive, adding 25 to 40 percent to the premium. Some companies using the automatic-increase approach charge a level premium for the inflation rider, while others increase the premium at the same rate as the benefit, which can make it prohibitively expensive.

Typically, insurers offer a choice of deductible periods after which benefits for policyholders begin. These periods can range from one to 365 days. In general, the shorter the deductible period, the higher the premium.

Long-term care insurance is expensive, even without inflation protection. A 65-year-old can expect to pay around $1,000 a year for both nursing home and home care coverage without inflation protection. Home care policies, by themselves, are less expensive, ranging from approximately $250 to $700 a year for a 65-year-old. And although all long-term care policies are guaranteed renewable, the rates you pay are not guaranteed to stay consistent. Most policies have level premiums that don't rise with the policyholder's age. However, if a carrier experiences more claims than expected, rates can rise across the board for all policyholders.

Another area to be concerned about is the financial stability of the company you purchase your policy from. Even companies rated highly can become insolvent, leaving policyholders with canceled policies or delays in getting their claims paid. Check with your state insurance department to see if they rate the financial strength of insurance companies. Similar information is available in your local library in the ratings published by Standard & Poor's and A.M. Best.

Tip

It is smart to check with your state insurance department to see if they rate the financial strength of insurance companies.

If you think long-term insurance, despite its wrinkles, is for you, here are some points and suggestions to consider. Unless you have a crystal ball to tell you what your future needs might be, it is best to buy a comprehensive insurance package that pays for both nursing home care and home care. Look for a policy that covers a wide range of services, with the least restrictions and no room for misinterpretation. While it may seem like a good idea to skip inflation protection because of its costs, don't. A year's stay in a nursing home in the year 2010 is expected to cost close to $80,000. A typical policy that pays $80 a day with no inflation protection would pay only around $30,000 of the bill, leaving $50,000 of uncovered expenses. You should also check with your state insurance department to see if it has a guaranty fund to take care of policyholders of insolvent companies in the event that your insurer folds. Also ask whether or not this fund, if it exists, covers policyholders who purchase plans from out-of-state companies.

Tip

It is best to buy a comprehensive insurance package that pays for both nursing home care and home care.

Shop carefully; only you can decide which policy, if any, suits you best.

Medical Emergencies

Chapter 27

One time you may not be able to choose a hospital is when you are involved in an emergency. When getting to the right hospital is most critical, your choice may be difficult to implement. The key to success is advance planning. For the most part, once an emergency occurs, it's out of your control.

Emergency response systems vary greatly by community. Until recent years, even in sophisticated medical communities, emergency medical systems were noted for their lack of coordination. Recently, a good deal of time and money have been spent on both state and local levels to improve these systems, but in many areas they are still fragmented, and the organization and delivery vary greatly.

Planning for an emergency should begin at home and be based on personal need, especially if some member of the family has a serious medical condition. Develop a family emergency response plan. Check the nearest hospital to be sure the emergency room (ER) is staffed 24 hours a day with physicians certified in emergency medicine. (While the term emergency department is coming into wide use in hospitals, this book uses the familiar ER.) Some hospitals staff ERs with any physicians they can find, regardless of specialty, including psychiatrists or other specialists who may not be well suited to this work. Other hospitals use doctors trained in medicine or surgery. While this is not the same as training in emergency medicine, these doctors may have had some continuing education in emergency medicine and, in general, are adequately prepared. In addition, hospitals should have nurses certified in emergency nursing. If you are satisfied that the hospital has the proper staff to respond to an emergency, you will feel safe specifying that hospital in your family response plan. If you do not feel the ER is well staffed, seek out another hospital. If you have an emergency in the home, you want to know in advance where you want to be treated. (It's a good idea to repeat this procedure for work sites as well.)

Emergency response systems vary greatly by community. Until recent years, even in sophisticated medical communities, emergency medical systems were noted for their lack of coordination.

The One, Two, Three of Emergency Preparations

There are three things a family should be aware of in an emergency:

- The 911 number is a universal number for emergency calls in many, but not all communities. Each call should be handled by a dispatcher who, based on the information available, decides if the response should be medical, police, or fire, or a combination. An *enhanced* 911 system reveals the location of the phone being used to make the call.
- Know which ambulance services will respond to an emergency medical call and assess them by the criteria described in the following pages. You will

often be able to use a particular service if a number of them serve your area and you call one in advance. You should also make certain your street name and house or apartment number are visible so you can be located easily.

- Be certain you have your family doctor's number close by. Your primary care doctor can help make sure your care is well coordinated by a visit or a call to the hospital. Obviously, a critical aspect of planning for emergencies involves whether or not your local Emergency Medical Service (EMS) is able to follow your directions. In most emergencies you can ask to be taken to a particular hospital (if you are able to communicate), and the emergency medical technician (EMT) will usually accede to your request if the hospital is within a reasonable distance (10 minutes is a good guide). The EMTs will make this decision based on your condition and will consider whether transportation to a more distant hospital would have an adverse effect. If the EMTs feel you need special care, however, as with burns or other serious trauma, they will bring you to a designated center. Another exception is heart attacks, in which the fastest stabilization possible is the basic goal, and you will very likely be brought to the closest ER. However, once a patient is stabilized, steps may be taken for transfer to a preferred hospital.

How Good Is Your EMS?

The following is a model that will be useful in assessing a local EMS. It is an ideal and probably does not exist in any single community, but it outlines the level of response and quality of care you should be seeking.

- Make sure that all emergency medical dispatchers are certified (in many communities they are not). A certified dispatcher is better trained to assess problems and talk people through emergency procedures such as administering CPR (cardiopulmonary resuscitation).
- Ask if dispatches are made on medical priority rather than on a first-come, first-served basis. If you're having a heart attack you do not want an ambulance to pick up someone with a sprained ankle just because they called first. (There is some resistance to this concept since communities are worried about liability if a dispatcher makes a miscall.)
- Be certain the first responders (often firefighters or police) have the appropriate medical training (50 hours or so) and are equipped with automatic defibrillators. Other personnel who might respond are EMS technicians (100 hours), and paramedics (1,000 hours). The better the responding team's training, the better a patient's chances for survival. While police, firefighters, and emergency medical technicians with less training than paramedics can clear air passages and use defibrillators, paramedics are the only emergency personnel allowed to administer drugs to support cardiac function or intubate to assist breathing. (EMTs are legally classed by level, i.e., 1, 2, 3, 4, and 5. The term paramedic refers to the highest level of training.)
- Ask if the system is headed by a professional with training and experience in pre-hospital medicine.

(An emergency response is only the first step in a continuum that includes pre-hospital emergency and inpatient or outpatient care.) Also ask about medical control and quality assurance. It is difficult for an untrained person to judge these factors, but at least make certain there are procedures in place.

- Ask if the siren and lights are used only when medically required. (A screaming siren can be upsetting to patients, family, and bystanders.)
- If a 911 system is in place, ask if it is enhanced. This is very important if the caller is disoriented, unable to communicate, does not speak English, or is a child.
- Ask if the system is accredited by the Commission on Accreditation of Ambulance Services (see Appendix N).

Remember, the response time of an emergency system depends on the information the dispatcher has, so it is important to supply accurate and complete information about the ill or injured person as well as a clear address, cross street, and landmarks.

If you ask all these questions and the responses leave you concerned about your emergency medical system, call the public officials responsible as well as local political leaders and urge that the system be improved. Public advocacy can support EMS leadership in obtaining the funds necessary to upgrade their systems. Emergency medical systems have been greatly improved in recent years, but much still remains to be done. As an informed consumer, you can help bring this change about and improve your own health care in the process. The American Ambulance Association is a good source of information on emergency medical systems (see Appendix N).

Tip

Remember, the response time of an emergency system depends on the information the dispatcher has, so it is important to supply accurate and complete information about the ill or injured person as well as a clear address, cross street, and landmarks.

In the ER

When you enter an ER you should expect to be treated according to the seriousness of your injuries or illness. The term used to describe this process is "triage," which comes from the French word triere, meaning "to part." Very simply, triage ensures that the sickest or most seriously injured patients are seen first, so you may have to wait unless your problem is critical. If you don't have life-threatening illness or injury, a wait of an hour or longer is not unusual.

Emergency departments are not designed to deliver primary care. Use your doctor or a free-standing clinic for non-emergency care.

Waiting time in a busy urban ER may also be quite different from a suburban ER. If there is a major fire, automobile accident, shootout, or if it's Saturday night (which is the busiest time in many ERs), an ER could be loaded with patients in critical condition. An executive or professional from an affluent suburb may think a half-hour wait is excessive, while an inner-city resident may feel an hour or two is a pretty quick response time. In many ERs four hours is a typical wait.

Obviously, you expect skilled, responsive care in an ER, and with today's specially trained doctors, nurses, and technicians, you may get it (chances are fifty-fifty!). A well-run emergency department should also provide privacy and cleanliness.

Emergencies Away from Home

> ***Tip***
>
> *You should receive good instructions on follow-up care when you leave the ER (assuming you're not hospitalized) and, if you don't have your own doctor, you can be referred to one.*

It is wise to prepare in advance for medical emergencies that could occur when traveling. If you are at risk—for example, if you have a serious heart condition—it is also a good idea to be sure your hotels have a medical emergency response capability. Many hotels have trained EMTs on staff and keep equipment such as defibrillators on hand. It can be well worth the few seconds it takes to check this out. Remember also, Medicare is not in effect overseas. If you are covered by Medicare you should make other health insurance arrangements.

There are a number of services available to assist travelers in need of medical care which can be found in Appendix L.

Carry a card that lists your blood type and other vital medical information such as allergies, current medications, chronic illnesses (e.g., diabetes, epilepsy), surgical history, next of kin, and insurance information, and the name and phone number of your primary care doctor. Make sure the card is filled out legibly and enclosed in plastic.

Tip

Carry a card that lists your blood type and other vital medical information such as allergies, current medications, chronic illnesses (e.g., diabetes, epilepsy), surgical history, next of kin, and insurance information, and the name and phone number of your primary care doctor. Make sure the card is filled out legibly and enclosed in plastic.

A medical alert tag, which can be worn around the neck or wrist, is also helpful. Vital information and critical medications can be inscribed on these tags, which are available from the Medic Alert Foundation (see Appendix L). Individuals can become members for an initial fee as low as $35 for which they receive a tag and have their medical histories filed with the foundation. The tag or bracelet carries vital information (e.g., medications, pacemakers) and a number that can be called 24 hours a day to obtain a computerized medical history. There is a $15 charge each year for maintaining and updating the information.

Also, carry all medications in their original containers when traveling. The prescription label can be extremely helpful in identifying medications in an emergency. You may also wish to carry an organ donor authorization card. To obtain an organ donation card, contact your local hospital.

An additional point: To avoid illness while traveling,

it is wise to receive complete immunizations recommended for the area to which you are traveling. Many hospitals, especially academic medical centers, offer such programs. Also, the Centers for Disease Control and Prevention offers a free fax line that will provide information on disease risks posed in different areas of the world, and will suggest appropriate precautions (see Appendix N).

Tip

The Centers for Disease Control and Prevention offers a free fax line that will provide information on disease risks posed in different areas of the world, and will suggest appropriate precautions.

If you are traveling and you need a doctor for a non-emergency, it is a good idea to call a major teaching hospital and ask for the chief resident of the appropriate service (e.g., internal medicine, ophthalmology, obstetrics & gynecology, etc.) and ask for a recommendation.

To find a doctor overseas, two US based services are available. International SOS Assistance finds English-speaking doctors, monitors your care and, if necessary, arranges transportation back to the US.

IAMAT, the International Association for Medical Assistance to Travelers, maintains a directory of English-speaking doctors whose credentials have been screened and who agree to a pre-set fee for treating IAMAT members. (See appendix L).

Appendixes

Patient's Bill of Rights
Appendix A

Your Rights in the Hospital

The American Hospital Association has adopted this Code of Patient Rights for hospitals to voluntarily observe:

1. The patient has a right to considerate and respectful care.

2. The patient has the right to and is encouraged to obtain from physicians and other direct caregivers relevant, current and understandable information concerning diagnosis, treatment and prognosis.

   Except in emergencies when the patient lacks decision-making capacity and the need for treatment is urgent, the patient is entitled to the opportunity to discuss and request information related to the specific procedures and/or treatments, the risks involved, the possible length of recuperation, and the medically reasonable alternatives and their accompanying risks and benefits.

   Patients have the right to know the identity of physicians, nurses and others involved in their care, as well as when those involved are students, residents or other trainees. The patient also has the right to know the immediate and long-term financial implications of treatment choices, insofar as they are known.

3. The patient has a right to make decisions about the plan of care prior to and during the course of treatment and to refuse a recommended treatment or plan of care to the extent permitted by law and hospital policy and to be informed of the medical consequences of this action. In case of such refusal, the patient is entitled to other appropriate care and services that the hospital provides or transfer to another hospital. The hospital should notify patients of any policy that might affect patient choice within the institution.

4. The patient has the right to have an advance directive

(such as a living will, health care proxy, or durable power of attorney for health care) concerning treatment or designating a surrogate decision maker with the expectation that the hospital will honor the intent of that directive to the extent permitted by law and hospital policy.

Health care institutions must advise patients of their rights under state law and hospital policy to make informed medical choices, ask if the patient has an advance directive, and include that information in patient records. The patient has the right to timely information about hospital policy that may limit its ability to implement fully a legally valid advance directive.

5. The patient has the right to every consideration of privacy. Case discussion, consultation, examination, and treatment should be conducted so as to protect each patient's privacy.

6. The patient has the right to expect that all communications and records pertaining to his/her care will be treated as confidential by the hospital, except in cases such as suspected abuse and public health hazards when reporting is permitted or required by law. The patient has the right to expect that the hospital will emphasize the confidentiality of this information when it releases it to any other parties entitled to review information in these records.

7. The patient has the right to review the records pertaining to his/her medical care and to have the information explained or interpreted as necessary, except when restricted by law.

8. The patient has the right to expect that, within its capacity and policies, a hospital will make reasonable response to the request of a patient for appropriate and medically indicated care and services. The hospital must provide evaluation, service and/or referral as indicated by the urgency of the case. When medically appropriate and legally permissible, or when a patient has so requested, a patient may be transferred to another facility. The institution to which the patient is to be

transferred must first have accepted the patient for transfer. The patient must also have the benefit of complete information and explanation concerning the need for risks, benefits and alternatives to such a transfer.

9. The patient has the right to ask and be informed of the existence of business relationships among the hospital, educational institutions, other health care providers, or payers that may influence the patient's treatment and care.

10. The patient has the right to consent or to decline to participate in proposed research studies or human experimentation affecting care and treatment or requiring direct patient involvement, and to have those studies fully explained prior to consent. A patient who declines to participate in research or experimentation is entitled to the most effective care that the hospital can otherwise provide.

11. The patient has the right to expect reasonable continuity of care when appropriate and to be informed by physicians and other caregivers of available and realistic patient care options when hospital care is no longer appropriate.

12. The patient has the right to be informed of hospital policies and practices that relate to patient care, treatment and responsibilities. The patient has the right to be informed of available resources for resolving disputes, grievances, and conflicts, such as ethics committees, patient representative or other mechanisms available in the institution. The patient has the right to be informed of the hospital's charges for services and available payment methods.

Hippocratic Oath Appendix B

The Hippocratic Oath is administered to all medical students when they graduate from their respective medical schools. Today, some Deans of Medicine administer it to their students as they enter medical school in order to instill in them a sense of ethics because even as students they will have contact with patients.

The oath is attributed to Hippocrates, a Greek physician who is often referred to as the Father of Medicine. Hippocrates advanced medical practice and ethics. He died circa 377 B.C.

The oath has been modified by various medical schools and professional bodies and will be found in a variety of forms that typically embody the same principles.

Hippocratic Oath. [Hippocrates. Greek physician, 460-377 B.C.] An oath setting forward the duties of a physician to his patients as follows:

I swear by Apollo the physician, and Asklepios, and health, and All-Heal and all the gods and goddesses, that, according to my ability and judgement, I will keep this Oath and this stipulation—to reckon him who taught me this Art equally dear to me as my parents, to share my substance with him, and relieve his necessities if required; to look upon his offspring in the same footing as my own brothers, and to teach them this Art, if they should wish to learn it, without fee or stipulation; and that by precept, lecture and every other mode of instruction, I will impart a knowledge of the Art to my own sons, and those of my teachers, and to disciples bound by a stipulation and oath according to the law of medicine, but to none others.

I will follow that system of regimen which, according to my ability and judgement, I consider for the benefit of my patients, and abstain from whatever is deleterious and mischievous, I will give no deadly medicine to anyone if asked nor suggest any such counsel; and in like manner I will not give to a woman a pessary to produce abortion. With purity and wholeness I will pass my life and practice my Art.

I will not cut persons laboring under the stone, but will leave this to be done by men who are practitioners of this work. Into whatever houses I enter, I will go into them for the benefit of the sick, and will abstain from every voluntary act of mischief and corruption; and, further, from the seduction of females or males, of freemen and slaves. Whatever, in connection with my professional practice, or not in connection with it, I see or hear, in the life of men, which ought not to be spoken of abroad, I will not divulge, as reckoning that all such should be kept secret. While I continue to keep this Oath unviolated, may it be granted to me to enjoy life and the practice of the art, respected by all men, in all times! But should I trespass and violate this Oath, may the reverse be my lot!

Dorland's Illustrated Medical Dictionary, 27th ed. W.B. Saunders Co., Philadelphia, 1988.

ABMS Approved Specialty Medical Boards Appendix C

24 Boards, 25 Specialties
(Psychiatry and Neurology share one board)

The following American Board of Medical Specialties approved medical specialty boards are responsible for the approval of the residency programs for training residents in a specialty and for the continuing certification of physicians in the specialty. Recertification periods and subspecialties are also listed.

To find out if a physician is certified, do not call the board. Call the ABMS at (708) 491-9091

Specialty Certification:	**Allergy and Immunology**
Subspecialty(ies):	Diagnostic Laboratory Immunology
Recertification:	Certifications awarded since 1989 are valid for 10 years. For those certified prior to 1989 there is no recertification requirement.
Address:	American Board of Allergy & Immunology University City Science Center 3624 Market Street Philadelphia, PA 19104 215-349-9466

Specialty Certification:	**Anesthesiology**
Subspecialty(ies):	Critical Care Medicine Pain Management
Recertification:	Presently, there is no recertification process.
Address:	American Board of Anesthesiology 100 Constitution Plaza Hartford, CT 06103 203-522-9857

Specialty Certification:	**Colon & Rectal Surgery**
Subspecialty(ies):	None
Recertification:	Presently there is no recertification process.
Address:	American Board of Colon and Rectal Surgery Heritage Bank Building 20600 Eureka Road, Suite 713 Taylor, MI 48108 313-282-9400
Specialty Certification:	**Dermatology**
Subspecialty(ies):	Dermatopathology Derm Immun/Diag Lab Immun Cutaneous Micrographic Surgery & Oncology
Recertification:	Certifications awarded since 1991 are valid for 10 years. For those certified prior to 1991, there is no recertification requirement.
Address:	American Board of Dermatology Henry Ford Hospital 2799 West Grand Boulevard Detroit, MI 48202 313-874-1088
Specialty Certification:	**Emergency Medicine**
Subspecialty(ies):	Pediatric Emergency Medicine Sports Medicine
Recertification:	Certifications are valid for a 10-year period.
Address:	American Board of Emergency Medicine 3000 Coolidge Road East Lansing, MI 48823 517-332-4800

Specialty Certification:	**Family Practice**
Subspecialty(ies):	Geriatric Medicine Sports Medicine
Recertification:	Certifications are valid for a 7-year period.
Address:	American Board of Family Practice 2228 Young Drive Lexington, KY 40505 606-269-5626

Specialty Certification:	**Internal Medicine**
Subspecialty(ies):	Adolescent Medicine Cardiac Electrophysiology Cardiovascular Disease Critical Care Medicine Diagnostic Laboratory Immunology Endocrinology & Metabolism Gastroenterology Geriatric Medicine Hematology Infectious Disease Medical Oncology Nephrology Pulmonary Disease Rheumatology Sports Medicine
Recertification:	Certifications awarded since 1990 are valid for 10 years. For those certified prior to 1990 there is no recertification requirement.
Address:	American Board of Internal Medicine University City Science Center 3624 Market Street Philadelphia, PA 19104 215-243-1500

Specialty Certification:	**Medical Genetics**
Subspecialty(ies):	None
Recertification:	Presently, there is no recertification requirement.
Address:	American Board of Medical Genetics 9650 Rockville Pike Bethesda, MD 20814 301-571-1825
Specialty Certification:	**Neurological Surgery**
Subspecialty(ies):	Critical Care Medicine
Recertification:	Presently, there is no recertification requirement.
Address:	American Board of Neurological Surgery Smith Tower, Suite 2139 6550 Fannin Street Houston, TX 77030-2701 713-790-6015
Specialty Certification:	**Nuclear Medicine**
Subspecialty(ies):	Nuclear Radiology Radioisotopic Pathology
Recertification:	Certifications awarded since 1992 are valid for 10 years. For those certified prior to 1992 there is no recertification requirement.
Address:	American Board of Nuclear Medicine 900 Veteran Avenue, Room 12-200 Los Angeles, CA 90024-1786 310-825-6787
Specialty Certification:	**Obstetrics & Gynecology**
Subspecialty(ies):	Critical Care Medicine Gynecologic Oncology Maternal & Fetal Medicine Reproductive Endocrinology

Recertification: Certifications awarded since 1986 are valid for 10 years. For those certified prior to 1992 there is no recertification requirement.

Address: American Board of Obstetrics and Gynecology
2915 Vine Street
Dallas, TX 75204
214-871-1619

Specialty Certification: Ophthalmology

Subspecialty(ies): None

Recertification: Certifications awarded since 1992 are valid for 10 years. For those certified prior to 1992 there is no recertification requirement.

Address: American Board of Ophthalmology
111 Presidential Boulevard, Suite 241
Bala Cynwyd, PA 19004
215-664-1175

Specialty Certification: Orthopaedic Surgery

Subspecialty(ies): Hand Surgery

Recertification: Certifications awarded since 1985 are valid for 10 years. For those certified prior to 1992 there is no recertification requirement.

Address: American Board of Orthopaedic Surgery
400 Silver Cedar Court
Chapel Hill, NC 27514
919-929-7103

Specialty Certification:	**Otolaryngology**
Subspecialty(ies):	Pediatric Otolaryngology
Recertification:	Presently, there is no recertification requirement.
Address:	American Board of Otolaryngology 5615 Kirby Drive, Suite 936 Houston, TX 77005 713-528-6200
Specialty Certification:	**Pathology**
Subspecialty(ies):	Blood Banking Chemical Pathology Cytopathology Dermatopathology Forensic Pathology Hematology Immunopathology Medical Microbiology Neuropathology Pediatric Pathology Radioisotopic Pathology
Recertification:	Presently, there is no recertification requirement.
Address:	American Board of Pathology Lincoln Center 5401 West Kennedy Boulevard PO Box 25915 Tampa, FL 33622-5915 813-286-2444
Specialty Certification:	**Pediatrics**
Subspecialty(ies):	Adolescent Medicine Pediatric Cardiology Pediatric Critical Care Medicine Diagnostic Laboratory Immunology Pediatric Gastroenterology Pediatric Infectious Disease Pediatric Endocrinology Pediatric Hematology-Oncology Pediatric Nephrology Pediatric Emergency Medicine

	Pediatric Pulmonology Neonatal-Perinatal Medicine Pediatric Rheumatology Pediatric Sports Medicine
Recertification:	Certifications awarded since 1988 are valid for 7 years. For those certified prior to 1988 there is no recertification requirement.
Address:	American Board of Pediatrics 111 Silver Cedar Court Chapel Hill, NC 27514-1651 919-929-0461
Specialty Certification:	**Physical Medicine and Rehabilitation**
Subspecialty(ies):	None
Recertification:	None
Address:	American Board of Physical Medicine and Rehabilitation Norwest Center, Suite 674 First Street, SW Rochester, MN 55902 507-282-1776
Specialty Certification:	**Plastic Surgery**
Subspecialty(ies):	Hand Surgery
Recertification:	Presently, there is no recertification requirement.
Address:	American Board of Plastic Surgery Seven Penn Center, Suite 400 1635 Market Street Philadelphia, PA 19103-2204 215-587-9322

Specialty Certification: **Preventive Medicine**
Subspecialty(ies): Underseas Medicine
Recertification: Presently, there is no recertification requirement.
Address: American Board of Preventive Medicine
9950 West Lawrence Avenue, Suite 106
Sullivan Park, IL 60176
708-671-1750

Specialty Certification: **Psychiatry & Neurology**
Subspecialty(ies): Addiction Psychiatry
Child & Adolescent Psychiatry
Geriatric Psychiatry
Clinical Neurophysiology
Recertification: Certifications awarded as of 1994 are valid for 10 years. For those certified prior to 1994 there is no recertification requirement.
Address: American Board of Psychiatry & Neurology
500 Lake Cook Road, Suite 335
Deerfield, IL 60015
708-945-7900

Specialty Certification: **Radiology**
Subspecialty(ies): Nuclear Radiology
Recertification: Presently, there is no recertification requirement (except for Radiation Oncology where certifications awarded as of 1994 are valid for 10 years. For those certified prior to 1994 there is no recertification requirement.)
Address: American Board of Radiology
5255 East Williams Circle, Suite 6800
Tucson, AZ 85711
602-790-2900

Specialty Certification:	**Surgery**
Subspecialty(ies):	General Vascular Surgery Hand Surgery Pediatric Surgery Surgical Critical Care
Recertification:	Presently, there is no recertification requirement.
Address:	American Board of Surgery 1617 John F. Kennedy Boulevard, Suite 860 Philadelphia, PA 19103-1847 215-568-4000
Specialty Certification:	**Thoracic Surgery**
Subspecialty(ies):	None
Recertification:	Certifications awarded since 1975 are valid for 10 years. For those certified prior to 1975 there is no recertification requirement.
Address:	American Board of Thoracic Surgery One Rotary Center, Suite 803 Evanston, IL 60201 708-475-1520
Specialty Certification:	**Urology**
Subspecialty(ies):	None
Recertification:	Certifications awarded as of 1985 are valid for 10 years. For those certified prior to 1985 there is no recertification requirement.
Address:	American Board of Urology 31700 Telegraph Road, Suite 150 Bingham Farms, MI 48025 810-646-9720

Board-Certified Medical Specialists Appendix D

In prior appendixes we listed various approved medical specialties. Following is a description of the types of health problems that these specialists and subspecialists treat. (Selected list.)

Allergist/Immunologist

Certified by the American Board of Allergy and Immunology, an allergist/immunologist diagnoses and treats allergies, asthma, and skin problems such as hives and contact dermatitis.

Anesthesiologist

Certified by the American Board of Anesthesiology, an anesthesiologist dispenses anesthetics and monitors the condition and vital signs of patients undergoing surgery.

Colon and Rectal Surgeon

Certified by the American Board of Colon and Rectal Surgery, a colon and rectal surgeon surgically treats diseases of the intestinal tract, colon and rectum, anal canal, and perianal area.

Dermatology

Certified by the American Board of Dermatology, a dermatologist diagnoses and treats benign and malignant disorders of the skin, mouth, external genitalia, hair and nails, as well as a number of sexually transmitted diseases.

Emergency Physician

Certified by the American Board of Emergency Medicine, an emergency physician deals with acute-care problems such as those seen in emergency room situations.

Family Practitioner

Certified by the American Board of Family Practice, a

family practitioner deals with and oversees the total health care of individual patients and their family members. Family practitioners are more common in rural areas and may perform procedures more commonly performed by specialists (e.g., minor surgery).

Gynecologist

Certified by the American Board of Obstetrics & Gynecology, a gynecologist diagnoses and treats problems associated with the female reproductive organs.

Internist

Certified by the American Board of Internal Medicine, an internist diagnoses and nonsurgically treats diseases, especially those of adults. Internists may act as primary care specialists, highly trained family doctors, or they may subspecialize in specialties such as cardiology or nephrology.

Immunologist (See Allergist/Immunologist)

Medical Geneticist

Certified by the American Board of Medical Genetics, a medical geneticist is a physician or scientist who identifies the genetic causes of inherited diseases and ailments and prevents, when possible, their occurrence.

Neurologist

Certified by the American Board of Psychiatry and Neurology, a neurologist diagnoses and medically treats disorders of the brain, spinal cord, and nervous system.

Neurological Surgeon

Certified by the American Board of Neurological Surgery, a neurosurgeon performs surgery on the brain, spinal cord, and nervous system.

Nuclear Medicine Specialist

Certified by the American Board of Nuclear Medicine, a nuclear medicine specialist, working in either a laboratory or with patients, evaluates the functions of all the organs in the body and treats thyroid disease, benign and malignant tumors, and radiation exposure through the use of radioactive substances.

Obstetrician

Certified by the American Board of Obstetrics & Gynecology, an obstetrician deals with the medical aspects of and intervention in pregnancy and labor.

Ophthalmologist

Certified by the American Board of Ophthalmology, an ophthalmologist diagnoses and treats diseases of and injuries to the eye.

Orthopaedic Surgeon

Certified by the American Board of Orthopaedic Surgery, an orthopaedic surgeon operates to correct injuries which interfere with the form and function of the extremities, spine, and associated structures.

Otolaryngologist

Certified by the American Board of Otolaryngology, an otolaryngologist (also known as ENT specialist) explores and treats diseases in the interrelated areas of the ears, nose, and throat.

Pathologist

Certified by the American Board of Pathology, a pathologist diagnoses and monitors disease by means of information gathered by laboratory tests and microscopic examination of tissue, cells, and bodily fluids.

Pediatrician

Certified by the American Board of Pediatrics, a pediatrician diagnoses and treats diseases of childhood and monitors the growth, development, and well-being of preadolescents.

Physiatrist

Certified by the American Board of Physical Medicine & Rehabilitation, a physiatrist uses physical therapy and physical agents such as water, heat, light, electricity, and mechanical manipulations in the diagnosis, treatment, and prevention of disease and body disorders.

Plastic Surgeon

Certified by the American Board of Plastic Surgery, a plastic surgeon specializes in reconstructive and cosmetic surgery of the face and other body parts.

Preventive Medicine

Certified by the American Board of Preventive Medicine, a physician who specializes in preventive medicine focuses on health prevention and on the health of groups rather than individuals.

Proctologist (See Colon and Rectal Surgeon)

Psychiatrist

Certified by the American Board of Psychiatry and Neurology, a psychiatrist examines, treats, and prevents mental illness through the use of psychoanalysis and/or drugs.

Radiologist

Certified by the American Board of Radiology, a radiologist studies and uses various types of radiation, including X-rays, in the diagnosis and treatment of disease. Some radiologic techniques no longer use radioactive equipment (e.g., MRI and ultrasound).

Surgeon

Certified by the American Board of Surgery, a surgeon treats disease, injury, and deformity by surgical procedures.

Thoracic Surgeon

Certified by the American Board of Thoracic Surgery, a thoracic surgeon performs surgery on the heart, lungs, and chest area.

Urologist

Certified by the American Board of Urology, a urologist diagnoses and treats diseases of the genitals in men and disorders of the urinary tract and bladder in both men and women.

Subspecialties

Addiction Psychiatry

A subspecialty certified by the American Board of Psychiatry and Neurology, Addiction Psychiatry deals with habitual psychological and physiological dependence on a substance or practice which is beyond voluntary control.

Adolescent Medicine

A subspecialty certified by both the American Board of Internal Medicine and the American Board of Pediatrics, Adolescent Medicine involves the primary care treatment of adolescents and young adults.

Aerospace Medicine

A subspecialty certified by the American Board of Preventive Medicine, Aerospace Medicine involves the study of the effects that high altitudes (such as diminished concentration of oxygen or lack of gravity) and other air travel factors have on health and performance.

Blood Banking/Transfusion Medicine

A subspecialty certified by the American Board of Pathology, Blood Banking involves the typing and safe separation of blood into several components for transfusion into patients.

Cardiac Electrophysiology

A subspecialty certified by the American Board of Internal Medicine, Cardiac Electrophysiology is the study of the electrical responses of the heart.

Cardiovascular Medicine

A subspecialty certified by the American Board of Internal

Medicine, Cardiovascular Medicine involves the diagnosis and treatment of disorders of the heart, lungs, and blood vessels.

Chemical Pathology

A subspecialty certified by the American Board of Pathology, Chemical Pathology involves the diagnosis of disease and injury related to chemical interactions in bodily tissues and cells.

Child & Adolescent Psychiatry

A subspecialty certified by the American Board of Psychiatry and Neurology, Child & Adolescent Psychiatry deals with the diagnosis and treatment of mental diseases in children and adolescents.

Clinical Cardiac Electrophysiology

A subspecialty certified by the American Board of Internal Medicine, Clinical Cardiac Electrophysiology involves complicated technical procedures to evaluate heart rhythms and determine appropriate treatment for them.

Clinical Neurophysiology

A subspecialty certified by the American Board of Psychiatry and Neurology, Clinical Neurophysiology is the study of the makeup and functioning of the nervous system in patients as opposed to in a laboratory.

Critical Care Medicine

A subspecialty certified by the American Boards of Anesthesiology, Internal Medicine, Neurological Surgery, and Obstetrics & Gynecology, a Critical Care specialist is required to diagnose and take immediate action to prevent death or further injury of a patient. Examples of critical injuries include shock, heart attack, drug overdose, and massive bleeding.

Cutaneous Micrographic Surgery & Oncology

A subspecialty certified by the American Board of

Pathology, Cytopathology is concerned with the study and diagnosis of health and disease by microscopic examination and evaluation of cellular specimens.

Dermatopathology

A subspecialty certified by both the American Board of Dermatology and the American Board of Pathology. Dermatopathology involves the evaluation of tissue specimens submitted from dermatologic patients on a cellular level through the examination and interpretation of microscopic slides of thin tissue sections and smears and scrapings from lesions of skin and related tissues.

Diagnostic Laboratory Immunology/Dermatologic Immunology

A subspecialty certified by the American Boards of Allergy & Immunology, Internal Medicine and Pediatrics, Diagnostic Laboratory Immunology refers to the testing process whereby the causes of immunity, induced sensitivity, and allergy are determined.

Endocrinology & Metabolism

A subspecialty certified by the American Board of Internal Medicine, Endocrinology & Metabolism involves the study and treatment of patients suffering from hormonal and chemical disorders.

Forensic Pathology

A subspecialty certified by the American Board of Pathology, Forensic Pathology deals with the diagnosis of the cause of death via information gathered through laboratory tests and microscopic examination of tissues, cells, and bodily fluids for use in legal proceedings.

Gastroenterology

A subspecialty certified by the American Board of Internal Medicine, Gastroenterology is the study, diagnosis and treatment of diseases of the digestive organs including the stomach, bowels, liver, and gallbladder.

General Vascular Surgery

A subspecialty certified by the American Board of Surgery, General Vascular Surgery involves the operative treatment of disorders of the blood vessels excluding those to the heart, lungs, or brain.

Geriatric Medicine

A subspecialty certified by the American Boards of Family Practice and Internal Medicine, Geriatric Medicine deals with diseases of the elderly and the problems associated with aging.

Geriatric Psychiatry

A subspecialty certified by the American Board of Psychiatry and Neurology, Geriatric Psychiatry involves the diagnosis, prevention, and treatment of mental illness in the elderly.

Gynecologic Oncology

A subspecialty certified by the American Board of Obstetrics and Gynecology, Gynecologic Oncology deals with cancers of the female genital tract and reproductive systems.

Hand Surgery

A subspecialty certified by the American Boards of Orthopaedic Surgery, Plastic Surgery, and Surgery, Hand Surgery involves the treatment of injury to the hand through surgical techniques.

Hematology

A subspecialty certified by the American Boards of Internal Medicine and Pathology, Hematology involves the diagnosis and treatment of diseases and disorders of the blood, bone marrow, spleen, and lymph glands.

Immunopathology

A subspecialty certified by the American Board of Pathology, Immunopathology is the study of immune reactions associated with disease, which may or may not result in a harmful clinical disorder.

Infectious Disease

A subspecialty certified by the American Board of Internal Medicine, Infectious Disease is the study and treatment of diseases caused by a bacterium, virus, fungus, or animal parasite. AIDS is an infectious disease.

Maternal & Fetal Medicine

A subspecialty certified by the American Board of Obstetrics and Gynecology, Maternal & Fetal Medicine involves the care of women with high-risk pregnancies and their unborn infants.

Medical Microbiology

A subspecialty certified by the American Board of Pathology, Medical Microbiology is the study of the effect of bacteria, fungi, viruses, and other microorganisms on human health.

Medical Oncology

A subspecialty certified by the American Board of Internal Medicine, Medical Oncology refers to the study and treatment of tumors and other cancers.

Neonatal-Perinatal Medicine

A subspecialty certified by the American Board of Pediatrics, Neonatal-Perinatal Medicine involves the diagnosis and treatment of infants prior to, during, and one month beyond birth.

Nephrology

A subspecialty certified by the American Board of Internal Medicine, Nephrology is concerned with disorders of the kidneys, high blood pressure, fluid and mineral balance, dialysis of body wastes when the kidneys do not function, and consultation with surgeons about kidney transplantation.

Neuropathology

A subspecialty certified by the American Board of Pathology, Neuropathology is the study of diseases of the nervous system as reflected in an altered structure.

Nuclear Radiology

A subspecialty certified by the American Boards of Nuclear Medicine and Radiology, Nuclear Radiology involves the use of radioactive substances to diagnose and treat certain functions and diseases of the body.

Occupational Medicine

A subspecialty certified by the American Board of Preventive Medicine, Occupational Medicine concentrates on the effects of the work environment on the health of employees.

Pediatric Cardiology

A subspecialty certified by the American Board of Pediatrics, Pediatric Cardiology involves the diagnosis and treatment of heart disease in children.

Pediatric Critical Care Medicine

A subspecialty certified by the American Board of Pediatrics, Pediatric Critical Care Medicine involves the care of children who are victims of life threatening disorders such as severe accidents, shock, and diabetes acidosis.

Pediatric Emergency Medicine

A subspecialty certified by both the American Boards of Emergency Medicine and Pediatrics, Pediatric Emergency Medicine refers to the treatment of children in an acute-care situation.

Pediatric Endocrinology

A subspecialty certified by the American Board of Pediatrics, Pediatric Endocrinology involves the study and treatment of children with hormonal and chemical disorders.

Pediatric Gastroenterology

A subspecialty certified by the American Board of Pediatrics, Pediatric Gastroenterology is the study, diagnosis, and treatment of diseases of the digestive tract in children.

Pediatric Hematology-Oncology

A subspecialty certified by the American Board of Pediatrics, Pediatric Hematology-Oncology is the study and treatment of cancers of the blood and blood-forming parts of the body in children.

Pediatric Infectious Disease

A subspecialty certified by the American Board of Pediatrics, Pediatric Infectious Disease is the study and treatment of diseases caused by a virus, bacterium, fungus, or animal parasite in children.

Pediatric Nephrology

A subspecialty certified by the American Board of Pediatrics, Pediatric Nephrology deals with the diagnosis and treatment of disorders of the kidneys in children.

Pediatric Otolaryngology

A subspecialty certified by the American Board of Otolaryngology, Pediatric Otolaryngology involves the diagnosis and treatment of disorders of the ear, nose, and throat which affect children.

Pediatric Pathology

A subspecialty certified by the American Board of Pathology, Pediatric Pathology involves the diagnosis and monitoring of disease in children through information gathered by lab tests and microscopic examination of cells, tissues, and bodily fluids.

Pediatric Pulmonology

A subspecialty certified by the American Board of Pediatrics, Pediatric Pulmonology involves the diagnosis and treatment of diseases of the chest, lungs, and chest tissue in children.

Pediatric Rheumatology

A subspecialty certified by the American Board of Pediatrics, Pediatric Rheumatology involves the treatment of diseases of the joints and connective tissues in children.

Pediatric Sports Medicine

A subspecialty certified by the American Board of Pediatrics, Pediatric Sports Medicine involves the diagnosis and treatment of injuries to the bone or soft tissue (muscles, tendons, ligaments) in children as a result of participation in athletic activity.

Pediatric Surgery

A subspecialty certified by the American Board of Surgery, Pediatric Surgery treats disease, injury, or deformity in children through surgical techniques.

Public Health & General Preventive Medicine

A subspecialty certified by the American Board of Preventive Medicine, Public Health and General Preventive Medicine involves the investigation of the causes of epidemic disease and the prevention of a wide variety of acute and chronic illnesses.

Pulmonary Disease

A subspecialty certified by the American Board of Internal Medicine, Pulmonary Disease involves the diagnosis and treatment of diseases of the chest, lungs, and airways.

Radiation Oncology

A subspecialty certified by the American Board of Radiology, Radiation Oncology involves the use of radiant energy and isotopes in the study and treatment of disease, especially malignant cancer.

Reproductive Endocrinology

A subspecialty certified by the American Board of Obstetrics and Gynecology, Reproductive Endocrinology deals with the endocrine system (including the pituitary, thyroid, parathyroid, adrenal glands, placenta, ovaries, and testes) and how its failure relates to infertility.

Rheumatology

A subspecialty certified by the American Board of Internal Medicine, Rheumatology involves the treatment of diseases of the joints, muscles, bones, and tendons.

Sports Medicine

A subspecialty certified by the American Boards of Emergency Medicine, Family Practice, and Internal Medicine, Sports Medicine refers to the practice of an orthopaedist or other physician who specializes in injuries to bone or soft tissue (muscles, tendons, ligaments) caused by participation in athletic activity.

Surgical Critical Care

A subspecialty certified by the American Board of Surgery, Surgical Critical Care involves the specialized care in the management of the critically ill patient, particularly the trauma victim and postoperative patient in the emergency department, intensive care unit, trauma unit, burn unit, and other similar settings.

Underseas Medicine

A subspecialty certified by the American Board of Preventive Medicine, Underseas Medicine is the field that encompasses all aspects of physiological and medical problems and therapeutic applications of barometric pressure greater than sea level.

Osteopathic Medicine Specialty Boards Appendix E

American Osteopathic Association
142 E Ontario Street
Chicago, IL 60611
312-280-7445

GENERAL CERTIFICATION

American Osteopathic Board of Anesthesiology

- Anesthesiology
    - No time-limited certificates

American Osteopathic Board of Dermatology

- Dermatology
    - No time-limited certificates

American Osteopathic Board of Emergency Medicine

- Emergency Medicine
    - Beginning 1/1/94, 10-year certificates

American Osteopathic Board of Family Physicians

- Family Practice
    - No time-limited certificates

American Osteopathic Board of Internal Medicine

- Internal Medicine
    - Beginning 1/1/93, 10-year certificates

American Osteopathic Board of Neurology and Psychiatry

- Neurology
- Psychiatry
    - Beginning 1/1/96, 10-year certificates

American Osteopathic Board of Obstetrics and Gynecology

- Obstetrics and Gynecology
  - No time-limited certificates

American Osteopathic Board of Ophthalmology and Otorhinolaryngology

- Ophthalmology
  - No time-limited certificates
- Otorhinolaryngology
- Facial Plastic Surgery
- Otorhinolaryngology and Facial Plastic Surgery
  - No time-limited certificates

American Osteopathic Board of Orthopaedic Surgery

- Orthopaedic Surgery
  - Beginning 1/1/94, 10-year certificates

American Osteopathic Board of Pathology

- Laboratory Medicine
- Anatomic Pathology
- Anatomic Pathology and Laboratory Medicine
  - Beginning 1/1/95, 10-year certificates

American Osteopathic Board of Pediatrics

- Pediatrics
  - Beginning 1/1/95, 7-year certificates

American Osteopathic Board of Preventive Medicine

- Preventive Medicine/Aerospace Medicine
- Preventive Medicine/Occupational-Environmental Medicine
- Preventive Medicine/Public Health
  - Beginning 1/1/94, 10-year certificates

American Osteopathic Board of Proctology

- Proctology
  - No time-limited certificates

American Osteopathic Board of Radiology

- Diagnostic Radiology
- Radiation Oncology
    - No time-limited certificates

American Osteopathic Board of Rehabilitation Medicine

- Rehabilitation Medicine
    - Beginning 6/1/95, 7-year certificates

American Osteopathic Board of Special Proficiency in Osteopathic Manipulative Medicine

- Special Proficiency in Osteopathic Manipulative Medicine
    - Beginning 1/1/95, 10-year certificates

American Osteopathic Board of Surgery

- Surgery (general)
- Plastic and Reconstructive Surgery
- Thoracic Cardiovascular Surgery
- Urological Surgery
- General Vascular Surgery
    - No time-limited certificates

Self-Designated Medical Specialty Interest Groups Appendix F

This list of self-designated medical specialty groups was obtained from the American Board of Medical Specialties. However, it is important to point out that these groups are not recognized by the ABMS, the governing board for the 24 medical specialty boards.

The organizations listed below range from highly organized groups that are attempting to formalize training and certification in their field to informal groups interested in a particular aspect of medicine.

If you wish to obtain information from any of these groups, you will have to do some detective work. Because so many are informal, the location, phone, and mailing address may change frequently, depending on the person who is functioning as secretary or administrator.

To track down one of these groups you might call a nearby academic health center in your area to see if they have a faculty or staff member known to be involved in that particular specialty. To find the names of academic health centers in your region call the Association of Academic Health Centers at (202) 265-9600. If that fails, try your community hospital.

A

Abdominal Surgeons
Acupuncture Medicine
Addiction Medicine
Addictionology
Adolescent Psychiatry
Aesthetic Plastic Surgery
Alcoholism and other Drug Dependencies (AMASODD)
Algology (Chronic Pain)
Alternative Medicine
Ambulatory Anesthesia
Ambulatory Foot Surgery

Anesthesia
Arthroscopy (Board of North America)
Arthroscopic Surgery

B

Bariatric Medicine
Bionic Psychology

C

Chelation Therapy
Chemical Dependence
Clinical Chemistry
Clinical Ecology
Clinical Medicine and Surgery
Clinical Neurology
Clinical Neurophysiology
Clinical Neurosurgery
Clinical Nutrition
Clinical Orthopaedic Surgery
Clinical Pharmacology
Clinical Polysomnography
Clinical Psychiatry
Clinical Psychology
Clinical Toxicology
Cosmetic Plastic Surgery
Cosmetic Surgery
Council of Non-Board-Certified Physicians
Critical Care in Medicine and Surgery

D

Dermatology
Disability Evaluating Physicians

E

Electrodiagnostic Medicine
Electroencephalography
Electromyography and Electrodiagnosis
Environmental Medicine
Epidemology (College)
Eye Surgery

F

Facial Cosmetic Surgery
Facial Plastic and Reconstructive Surgery
Forensic Psychiatry
Forensic Toxicology

H

Hand Surgery
Head, Facial and Neck Pain and TMJ Orthopaedics
Health Physics
Homeopathic Physicians
Homeotherapeutics
Hypnotic Anesthesiology, National Board for Industrial Medicine and Surgery

I

Insurance Medicine
International Cosmetic and Plastic Facial Reconstructive Studies
Interventional Radiology

L

Laser Surgery
Law in Medicine
Longevity Medicine/Surgery

M

Malpractice Physicians
Maxillofacial Surgeons
Medical Accreditation (American Federation for)
Medical Hypnosis
Medical Laboratory Immunology
Medical-Legal Analysis of Medicine and Surgery
Medical-Legal Consultants
Medical, Legal and Workers Compensation
Medicine and Surgery
Medical Management
Medical Microbiology
Medical Preventics (Academy)
Medical Psychotherapists
Medical Toxicology
Microbiology (Medical Microbiology)
Military Medicine
Mohs Micrographic Surgery and Cutaneous Oncology

N

Neuroimaging
Neurologic and Orthopaedic Dental Medicine and Surgery
Neurological and Orthopaedic Medicine
Neurological and Orthopaedic Surgery
Neurological Microsurgery
Neurology
Neuromuscular Thermography
Neuro-Orthopaedic Dental Medicine and Surgery
Neuro-Orthopaedic Electrodiagnosis
Neuro-Orthopaedic Laser Surgery
Neuro-Orthopaedic Psychiatry
Neuro-Orthopaedic Thoracic Medicine/Surgery
Neurorehabilitation
Nutrition

O

Orthopaedic Medicine
Orthopaedic Microneurosurgery
Otorhinolaryngology

P

Pain Management (American Academy of)
Pain Management Specialties
Pain Management
Percutaneous Diskectomy
Plastic Esthetic Surgeons
Professional Disability Consultants Prison Medicine
Psychiatric Medicine
Psychiatry (National Board of)
Psychoanalysis (American Examining Board in)
Psychological Medicine (International)

Q

Quality Assurance and Utilization Review

R

Radiology and Medical Imaging
Rheumatologic and Reconstructive Medicine
Ringside Medicine and Surgery

S

Skin Specialists
Sleep Medicine (Polysomnography)
Spinal Cord Injury
Spinal Surgery
Sports Medicine
Sports Medicine/Surgery

T

Toxicology
Trauma Surgery
Traumatologic Medicine and Surgery
Tropical Medicine

U

Ultrasound Technology
Urological Surgery
Urologic Allied Health Professionals

W

Weight Reduction Medicine

State Agencies
Appendix G

While there is a wealth of information available through these state agencies, much of it is not user-friendly. Dense contractual agreements and other legal documents contain information that, could a consumer locate it, may prove to be very valuable. Often a department will suggest that a consumer visit the office for guidance in reviewing the documents.

Alabama

Doctors

Alabama Board of Medical Examiners
PO Box 946
Montgomery, AL 36101
Tel: 205-242-4116

Hospitals

Alabama Department of Public Health
Division of Licensure and Certification
434 Monroe Street
Montgomery, AL 36130
Tel: 205-240-3503

State Health and Planning Development Agencies
312 Montgomery Street, 7th Floor
Montgomery, AL 36104
Tel: 205-242-4103

HMOs

Alabama Department of Public Health
Bureau of Health Care Standards
Division of Planning and Program Development
434 Monroe Street
Montgomery, AL 36130
Tel: 205-613-5366

Department of Insurance
135 South Union Street
Montgomery, AL 36130
Tel: 205-269-3550

Alaska

Doctors

Alaska State Medical Association
4107 Laurel Street
Anchorage, AL 99508
Tel: 907-562-2662

Hospitals

Health Facility Certification and Licensing
4796-6 Business Park Boulevard
Building H
Anchorage, AL 99503
Tel: 907-561-8081

HMOs

Currently, there are no HMOs operating in Alaska.

Arizona

Doctors

Arizona Board of Medical Examiners
2001 West Camelback Road, Suite 300
Phoenix, AZ 85012
Tel: 602-255-3751

Hospitals

Arizona Dept. of Health Services
Division of EMS/Health Care Facilities,
Office of Health Care Licensure
100 West Clarendon, 4th Floor
Phoenix, AZ 85013
Tel: 602-255-1177

HMOs

Department of Insurance
2910 North 44th Street, Suite 210
Phoenix, AZ 85012
Tel: 602-912-8400

Arkansas

Doctors

Arkansas State Medical Board
2100 Riverfront Drive, Suite 200
Little Rock, AR 72202
Tel: 501-296-1802

Hospitals

Department of Health
Division of Health Facility Services
4815 West Markham Street, Mail Slot 9
Little Rock, AR 72205-3867
Tel: 501-661-2201

HMOs

Arkansas Insurance Department
400 University Tower Building
Little Rock, AR 72204
Tel: 501-686-2900

California

Doctors

California Medical Board
1426 Howe Avenue, Suite 54
Sacramento, CA 95825-3236
Tel: 916-263-2499

Hospitals

Licensing & Certification
Headquarters
1800 Third Street, Suite 210
PO Box 942732
Sacramento, CA 94234
Tel: 916-327-7015

Sacramento District	916-387-2500
Chico District	916-895-6711
Santa Rose District	707-576-2380
Berkeley District	310-540-2417
Daly City District	415-301-9971
San Jose District	408-277-1784
Fresno District	209-445-5168
Ventura District	805-654-4800
Orange County District	714-558-4001
San Diego District	619-688-6190
San Bernadino District	909-383-4777
Los Angeles County	213-351-8200

HMOs

Department of Corporations
Division of Healthcare Service Claims
1115 11th Street
Sacramento, CA 95814
Tel: 916-654-8076

Colorado

Doctors

Colorado Board of Medical Examiners
1560 Broadway, Suite 1300
Denver, CO 80202-5140
Tel: 303-894-7690

Hospitals

Department of Health
Department of Health Facilities
4300 Cherry Creek Drive South
Denver, CO 80222-15300
Tel: 303-692-2000

HMOs

Division of Insurance
1560 Broadway, Suite 850
Denver, CO 80202
Tel: 303-894-7499

Connecticut

Doctors

Department of Public Health and Administration
Licensure and Registration
150 Washington Street
Hartford, CT 06106
Tel: 203-566-5296

Department of Health Service
Hearing Office
150 Washington Street
Hartford, CT 06106
Tel: 203-566-1011

Hospitals

Connecticut State Department of Public Health &
Addiction Services
Division of Hospital and Medical Care
150 Washington Street
Hartford, CT 06106
Tel: 203-566-5758

HMOs

Department of Insurance
PO Box 816
153 Market Street, 11th Floor
Hartford, CT 06142
Tel: 203-297-3800

Commission of Hospitals and Health Care
1049 Asylum Avenue
Hartford, CT 06105
Tel: 203-566-3880

Delaware

Doctors

Board of Medical Practice of Delaware
Division of Professional Regulation
Margaret O'Neill Building, 2nd Floor
PO Box 1401
Dover, DE 19903
Tel: 302-739-4522

Hospitals

Department of Health Facilities Licensing and Certification
3 Mill Road, Suite 308
Wilmington, DE 19806
Tel: 302-577-6666

Peer Health Planning and Resources Management
Delaware Health Statistics Center
Jesse Cooper Building
PO Box 637
Dover, DE 19903
Tel: 302-739-4776

HMOs

Department of Insurance
841 Silver Lake Boulevard
Dover, DE 19901
Tel: 302-739-4251

District of Columbia

Doctors

District of Columbia Board of Medicine
Department of Consumer Affairs
605 G Street, Room 202LL
Washington, DC 20001
Tel: 202-727-5365 (M–F 9 AM–3 PM)

Hospitals

Occupational and Professional Licensing Administration
License & Certification Division
614 H Street, NW, Suite 931
Washington, DC 20001
Tel: 202-727-7823

HMOs

Department of Insurance Administration
441 4th Street, NW, 8th Floor North
Washington, DC 20001
Tel: 202-727-8000

Florida

Doctors

Florida Board of Medicine
1940 North Monroe Street
Tallahassee, FL 32399
Tel: 904-488-0595

Hospitals

Agency for Healthcare Administration
Hospital Unit
2727 Mahan Drive
Tallahassee, FL 32308
Tel: 904-487-2717

Agency for Healthcare Administration
Certificate of Need Office
2727 Mahan Drive
Tallahassee, FL 32308
Tel: 904-488-8673

Agency for Healthcare Administration
State Center for Health Statistics, Research & Analysis
325 John Knox Road
Atrium Building, Suite 301
Tallahassee, FL 32303
Tel: 904-922-5771

HMOs

Florida Department of Insurance
Bureau of Specialty Insurers
200 East Gaines Street
Tallahassee, FL 32399
Tel: 904-922-3131

Georgia

Doctors

Composite State Board of Medical Examiners
166 Pryor Street South West
Atlanta, GA 30303
Tel: 404-656-3913

Hospitals

Department of Human Resources
Office of Regulatory Services
Health Care Section
2 Peachtree Street, NW, 19th Floor
Atlanta, GA 30303
Tel: 404-657-5550

HMOs

Licensing Department
Georgia Department of Insurance
7th Floor, West Tower
2 Martin Luther King Drive
Atlanta, GA 30334
Tel: 404-656-2100

Hawaii

Doctors

Board of Medical Examiners
Professional Vocational Division
PO Box 3469
Honolulu, HI 96801
Tel: 808-586-3000

Regulated Industries Complaint Office
Licensing Division
PO Box 2399
Honolulu, HI 96804
Tel: 808-586-2677

Hospitals

Department of Health
Hospital and Medical Facilities
Medicare Section
1270 Queen Emma Street, Suite 1100
Honolulu, HI 96813
Tel: 808-586-4077

HMOs

Department of Health
Hospital and Medical Facilities
Medicare Section
1270 Queen Emma Street, Suite 1100
Honolulu, HI 96813
Tel: 808-586-4077

Idaho

Doctors

Idaho State Board of Medical Examiners
PO Box 83720
Boise, ID 83720-0058
Tel: 208-334-2822

Hospitals

Department of Health and Welfare
Bureau of Facility Standards, Licensing and Certification
Statehouse Mall
450 West State Street, 2nd Floor
Boise, ID 83720
Tel: 208-334-6626

Office of Health Policy and Resource Development
Division of Health
Idaho Department of Health and Welfare
450 West State Street, 4th Floor
Boise, ID 83720
Tel: 208-334-5992

HMOs

Department of Insurance
Division of Examination
700 West State Street
Boise, ID 83720
Tel: 208-334-2250

Illinois

Doctors

Illinois Department of Professional Regulation
320 West Washington Street, 3rd Floor
Springfield, IL 62786
Tel: 217-785-0820

Hospitals

Illinois Department of Public Health
535 West Jefferson Street
Springfield, IL 62761
Tel: 217-782-5750

Health Care Cost Containment
4500 South 6th Street Road
Springfield, IL 62703
Tel: 217-786-7001

HMOs

Illinois Department of Health
HMO Compliance Unit
320 West Washington Street
Springfield, IL 62767
Tel: 217-782-4515

Indiana

Doctors

Medical Licensing Board of Indiana
Health Professions Bureau
Records Division, Room 041
402 West Washington Street
Indianapolis, IN 46204
Tel: 317-233-4432

Department of Insurance
311 West Washington Street, Suite 300
Indianapolis, IN 46204
Tel: 317-232-5065/5430

Hospitals

Indiana State Department of Health
Division of Acute Care
1330 West Michigan Street, Room 336
Indianapolis, IN 46202
Tel: 317-633-8400

HMOs

Indiana Department of Insurance
311 West Washington Street, Suite 300
Indianapolis, IN 46204
Tel: 317-232-2385

Iowa

Doctors

Iowa State Board of Medical Examiners
State Capital Complex
Executive Hills West
Des Moines, IA 50319
Tel: 515-281-5171

Hospitals

Department of Inspections & Appeals
Health Facilities
Lucas State Office Building
Des Moines, IA 50319
Tel: 515-281-4115

HMOs

Division of Insurance
Lucas State Office Building
Des Moines, IA 50319
Tel: 515-281-5705

Kansas

Doctors

Kansas State Board of Healing Arts
235 South Topeka Boulevard
Topeka, KS 66603
Tel: 913-296-7413

Hospitals

Bureau of Adult & Child Care
Kansas Department of Health and Environment
Landon State Office Building, Suite 1001
900 SW Jackson
Topeka, KS 66612-1290
Tel: 913-296-1240

Kansas Dept. of Health & Environment
Research and Analysis Department
109 SW 9th Street
Mills Building, Suite 400 A
Topeka, KS 66612-2219
Tel: 913-296-5645

HMOs

Kansas Insurance Department
420 SW 9th Street
Topeka, KS 66612
Tel: 913-296-3071

Kentucky

Doctors

Kentucky Medical Licensure Board
310 Whittington Parkway, Suite 1B
Louisville, KY 40222
Tel: 502-429-8046

Hospitals

Division of Licensing and Regulation, Cabinet for Human Resources
CHR Building, 4th Floor
275 East Main Street
Frankfort, KY 40621
Tel: 502-564-2800

Division of Licensing and Regulation
Health Data Branch
275 East Main Street
Frankfort, KY 40621
Tel: 502-564-2757

HMOs

Division of Licensing and Regulation, Cabinet for Human Resources
CHR Building, 4th Floor
275 East Main Street
Frankfurt, KY 40621
Tel: 502-564-2800

Department of Insurance, Life and Health Division
215 West Main Street
PO Box 517
Frankfurt, KY 40602
Tel: 502-564-6088

Department of Insurance,
Financial Standards and Examination Division
215 West Main Street
PO Box 517
Frankfurt, KY 40602
Tel: 502-564-6082

Department of Insurance, Property and Casualty Division
215 West Main Street
Frankfurt, KY 40601
Tel: 502-564-3630

Louisiana

Doctors

Louisiana State Board of Medical Examiners
830 Union Street, Suite 100
New Orleans, LA 70112
Tel: 504-524-6763

Hospitals

Department of Health and Hospitals
Bureau of Health Services Financing,
Health Standards Section
PO Box 3767
Baton Rouge, LA 70821
Tel: 504-342-0138

HMOs

Department of Insurance
PO Box 94214
Baton Rouge, LA 70804-9214
Tel: 504-342-5900

Maine

Doctors

Board of Licensure and Medicine
2 Bangor Street
State House, Station 137
Augusta, ME 04333
Tel: 207-287-3601

Hospitals

Division of Licensing and Certification,
Department of Human Services
State House, Station 11
Augusta, ME 04333
Tel: 207-624-5443

HMOs

Bureau of Insurance
Department of Professional and Financial Regulation
State House, Station 34
Augusta, ME 04333
Tel: 207-582-8707

Maryland

Doctors

Board of Physician Quality Assurance
4201 West Patterson Avenue
Baltimore, MD 21215
Tel: 410-764-4777

Hospitals

Licensing and Certification Programs
4201 West Patterson Avenue
Baltimore, MD 21215
Tel: 410-764-2750

Health Services Cost Review Commission
4201 West Patterson Avenue
Baltimore, MD 21215
Tel: 410-764-2605

Maryland Health Resources Planning Commission
4201 West Patterson Avenue
Baltimore, MD 21215
Tel: 410-764-3255

HMOs

Department of Licensing and Regulation,
Insurance Division
501 St. Paul Place
Baltimore, MD 21202
Tel: 410-333-6300

Life and Health Section
Maryland Insurance Administration
501 St. Paul Place
Baltimore, MD 21202
Tel: 410-333-6104

Massachusetts

Doctors

Board of Registration in Medicine
10 West Street
Boston, MA 02111
Tel: 617-727-3086

Hospitals

Division of Health Care Quality
Dept. of Public Health
10 West Street, 5th Floor
Boston, MA 02111
Tel: 617-727-5860

Bureau of Health Statistics, Research and Evaluation
Massachusetts Department of Public Health
150 Tremont Street, 8th Floor
Boston, MA 02111
Tel: 617-727-6452

HMOs

Massachusetts Division of Insurance
490 Atlantic Avenue
Boston, MA 02201
Tel: 617-521-7777 (Consumer Help Line)

Michigan

Doctors

Michigan Board of Medicine
611 West Ottawa Street
Box 30018
Lansing, MI 48909
Tel: 517-373-6873

Hospitals

Division of Licensing and Certification
3500 North Logan Street
Lansing, MI 48909
Tel: 517-335-8505

Division of Licensing and Certification
PO Box 30195
3423 North Logan/Martin Luther King Jr. Boulevard
Lansing, MI 48909
Tel: 517-334-8408

HMOs

Department of Commerce Michigan Insurance Bureau
PO Box 30220
Lansing, MI 48909
Tel: 517-373-0240

Michigan Department of Public Health
3423 Martin Luther King Boulevard
Lansing, MI 48909
Tel: 517-335-8551

Minnesota

Doctors

Minnesota Board of Medical Practice
2700 University Avenue, W, Suite 106
St. Paul, MN 55114
Tel: 612-642-0538

Hospitals

Minnesota Department of Health
Health Resources Division
Central Medical Building
393 North Dunlap
PO Box 64900
St. Paul, MN 55164-0900
Tel: 612-643-2149

HMOs

Minnesota Department of Health
Occupational and Systems Compliance Division
Managed Care Systems Section
121 East 7th Place, Suite 400
St. Paul, MN 55101
Tel: 612-282-5614

Mississippi

Doctors

State Medical Licensure Board
2688 D Insurance Center Drive
Jackson, MS 39216
Tel: 601-354-6645

Hospitals

State Health Department
Division of Health Facility Licensure and Certification
PO Box 1700
Jackson, MS 39215
Tel: 601-354-7300

HMOs

State Health Department
Division Licensure & Certification
PO Box 1700
Jackson, MS 39215
Tel: 601-354-7300

Missouri

Doctors

Missouri State Board of Registration for the Healing Arts
3605 Missouri Boulevard, Box 4
Jefferson City, MO 65102
Tel: 314-751-0098

Department of Health
PO Box 570
Jefferson City, MO 65102
Tel: 314-751-6279

Hospitals

Bureau of Hospital Licensing and Certification
PO Box 570
Jefferson City, MO 65102
Tel: 314-751-6302

Department of Health
PO Box 570
Jefferson City, MO 65102
Tel: 314-751-6279

HMOs

Department of Insurance
PO Box 690
Jefferson City, MO 65101
Tel: 314-751-2640/800-726-7390

Montana

Doctors

Professional and Occupational Licensing
Board of Medical Examiners
111 North Jackson, Box 200513
Helena, MT 59620-0513
Tel: 406-444-4276

Hospitals

Bureau of Licensing and Certification
Health Facilities Division
WF Cogswell Building
Helena, MT 59620
Tel: 406-444-2676

Health Services Division
Health Planning Program
Cogswell Building, Room C216
Helena, MT 59620
Tel: 406-444-5268

HMOs

Insurance Department
PO Box 4009
Helena, MT 59604
Tel: 406-444-2040

Nebraska

Doctors

Bureau of Examining Boards
301 Centennial Mall South
Lincoln, NE 68509-5009
Tel: 402-471-2115

Hospitals

Department of Health
Bureau of Health Facilities Standards
301 Centennial Mall South
Lincoln, NE 68509-5007
Tel: 402-471-2946

HMOs

Department of Insurance
941 O Street, Suite 400
Lincoln, NE 68508
Tel: 402-471-2201

Nevada

Doctors

Nevada State Board of Medical Examiners
PO Box 7238
Reno, NV 89510
Tel: 702-688-2559

Hospitals

Bureau of Licensure and Certification,
Nevada Health Division
505 East King, Suite 202
Carson City, NV 89710
Tel: 702-687-4475

HMOs

Department of Business and Industry
Division of Insurance
1665 Hot Springs Road, Suite 152
Carson City, NV 89710
Tel: 702-687-4270

New Hampshire

Doctors

New Hampshire Board of Registration in Medicine
2 Industrial Park Drive, Suite 8
Concord, NH 03301-8520
Tel: 603-271-1203

Hospitals

Bureau of Health Facilities Administration
6 Hazen Drive
Concord, NH 03301
Tel: 603-271-4592

HMOs

Department of Insurance
169 Manchester Street
Concord, NH 03301
Tel: 603-271-2261

New Jersey

Doctors

Board of Medical Examiners
140 East Front Street
Trenton, NJ 08608
Tel: 609-826-7100

Hospitals

Department of Health
Division of Health Facilities Evaluation and Licensing
CN-367
Trenton, NJ 08625
Tel: 609-588-7725

HMOs

Department of Health
Division of Health Facilities Evaluation and Licensing
CN-367
Trenton, NJ 08625
Tel: 609-588-7725

Department of Health
Alternative Health Systems
CN-367
Trenton, NJ 08625
Tel: 609-588-2510

Department of Insurance
Division of Actuarial Services, Life and Health
Managed Healthcare Bureau
20 West State Street
CN-325
Trenton, NJ 08625
Tel: 609-984-8276

New Mexico

Doctors

New Mexico Board of Medical Examiners
491 Old Santa Fe Trail
Lamy Building, 2nd Floor
Santa Fe, NM 87501
Tel: 505-827-7317

Hospitals

Department of Health
Health Facility Licensing and Certification Bureau
525 Camino De Los Marquez, Suite 2
Santa Fe, NM 87501
Tel: 505-827-4200

Health Policy Commission
410 Don Gaspar
Santa Fe, NM 87501
Tel: 505-827-4488

HMOs

New Mexico Department of Insurance
PO Drawer 1269
Santa Fe, NM 87504-1269
Tel: 505-827-4500

New Mexico Department of Insurance
Consumer Division
PO Drawer 1269
Santa Fe, NM 87504-1269
Tel: 505-827-4500

New York

Doctors

New York State Department of Health
Corning Tower
Empire State Plaza
Albany, NY 12237
Tel: 518-474-8357

New York State Department of Education
Cultural Education Center
Division of Professional Licensing
Albany, NY 12230
Tel: 518-486-5205

Hospitals

Office of Health Systems Management
Tower Building
Empire State Plaza
Albany, NY 12237-0701
Tel: 518-474-7028

New York State Department of Health
Bureau of Biometrics
Concourse Room C-144
Empire State Plaza
Albany, NY 12237
Tel: 518-474-3189

HMOs

Department of Insurance
Health and Life Policy Bureau
Agency Building 1
Empire State Plaza
Albany, NY 12257
Tel: 518-474-4098

New York State Department of Health
Bureau of Alternative Delivery Systems
Corning Tower, Room 1911
Albany, NY 12237
Tel: 518-473-8944

New York State Department of Health
Bureau of Management Analysis
Records Access Office
Corning Tower, Room 2230
Albany, NY 12237
Tel: 518-474-8734

North Carolina

Doctors

North Carolina Board of Medical Examiners
PO Box 20007
Raleigh, NC 27609
Tel: 919-828-1212

Hospitals

Division of Facility Services
Licensure Section, Acute Care Branch
PO Box 29530
Raleigh, NC 27626-0530
Tel: 919-733-1604

Medical Database Commission
112 Cox Avenue
Raleigh, NC 27605
Tel: 919-733-7141

HMOs

Department of Insurance
Managed Care and Health Benefits Division
112 Cox Avenue
Raleigh, NC 27605
Tel: 919-715-0526

Department of Insurance
Financial Compliance Division
430 North Salisbury Street
Raleigh, NC 27603
Tel: 919-733-5633

Department of Insurance
Life and Health Division
430 North Salisbury Street
Raleigh, NC 27603
Tel: 919-733-5060

Department of Insurance
Consumer Services Division
PO Box 26387
Raleigh, NC 27611
Tel: 919-733-2004

North Dakota

Doctors

North Dakota State Board of Medical Examiners
City Center Plaza
418 East Broadway Avenue, Suite 12
Bismarck, ND 58505
Tel: 701-223-9485

Hospitals

Division of Health Facilities
North Dakota Department of Health
600 East Boulevard
Bismarck, ND 58505
Tel: 701-224-2352

HMOs

Department of Insurance
State Capitol
600 East Boulevard
Bismarck, ND 58505
Tel: 701-224-2440

Ohio

Doctors

State Medical Board of Ohio
77 South High Street, 17th Floor
Columbus, OH 43266-0315
Tel: 614-466-3934

Hospitals

Ohio Department of Health
Office of Resources Development
246 North High Street
Columbus, OH 43266-0588
Tel: 614-466-3325

Ohio Department of Health
Office of Health Policy
246 North High Street
Columbus, OH 43268-0588
Tel: 614-644-1912

HMOs

Department of Insurance
Managed Care Division
2100 Stella Court
Columbus, OH 43266-0566
Tel: 614-644-2661

Oklahoma

Doctors

Oklahoma State Board of Medical Licensure and Supervision
PO Box 18256
Oklahoma City, OK 73154-0256
Tel: 405-848-6841

Hospitals

State Department of Health
1000 NE 10th Street
Oklahoma City, OK 73117-1299
Tel: 405-271-6868

State Department of Health
Health Planning
1000 NE 10th Street
Oklahoma City, OK 73117-1299
Tel: 405-271-3943

HMOs

State Department of Health
Special Health Services
1000 NE 10th Street
Oklahoma City, OK 73117-1299
Tel: 405-271-6868

Oregon

Doctors

Board of Medical Examiners
1500 South West 1st Avenue, Suite 620
Portland, OR 97201-5826
Tel: 503-229-5770

Hospitals

Oregon Health Division
Health Care Licensing and Certification
PO Box 14450
Portland, OR 97214
Tel: 503-731-4013

Office of Health Policy
Suite 640
800 North East Oregon Street, #23
Portland, OR 97232
Tel: 503-731-4091

HMOs

Department of Consumer and Business Services
Insurance Division 440-4
Labor and Industries Building
Salem, OR 97310
Tel: 503-378-4271

Department of Consumer and Business Services
470 Labor and Industries Building
Salem, OR 97310-0700
Tel: 503-378-4481

Department of Consumer and Business Services
Attn: Consumer Advocacy
440 Labor and Industries Building
Salem, OR 97310-0700
Tel: 503-378-4484

Pennsylvania

Doctors

State Board of Medicine
PO 2649
Harrisburg, PA 17105
Tel: 717-783-1400

Hospitals

Division of Hospitals
Health and Welfare Building, Suite 532
Harrisburg, PA 17120
Tel: 717-783-8980

Pennsylvania Health Department
Division of Health Statistics and Research
State Center
PO Box 90
Harrisburg, PA 17108
Tel: 717-783-2548

HMOs

Department of Insurance
1321 Strawberry Square
Harrisburg, PA 17120
Tel: 717-787-2317 – (Consumer Services)

Department of Insurance
1345 Strawberry Square
Harrisburg, PA 17120
Tel: 717-787-5890

Department of Health
Bureau of Healthcare Financing
Room 1026, Health and Welfare Building
Box 90
Harrisburg, PA 17108
Tel: 717-787-5193

Department of Insurance
1400 Spring Garden Street, Room 1701
Philadelphia, PA 19130
Tel: 215-560-2630

Pennsylvania Insurance Department
300 Liberty Avenue
304 State Office Building
Pittsburgh, PA 15222
Tel: 412-565-5020

Erie Regional Office
Pennsylvania Insurance Department
Room 513 Baldwin Building
PO Box 6142
Erie, PA 16512
Tel: 814-871-4466

Rhode Island

Doctors

Rhode Island Department of Health
Rhode Island Board of Medical Licensure and Discipline
3 Capitol Hill
Providence, RI 02908
Tel: 401-277-3855

Hospitals

Rhode Island Department of Health
Division of Facilities Regulation
3 Capitol Hill
Providence, RI 02908
Tel: 401-277-2566

HMOs

Division of Insurance
Department of Business Regulation
233 Richmond Street, Suite 233
Providence, RI 02903
Tel: 401-277-2223

South Carolina

Doctors

State Board of Medical Examiners of South Carolina
101 Executive Center Drive
Saluda Building, Suite 120
PO Box 212269
Columbia, SC 29221-2269
Tel: 803-731-1650

Hospitals

Department of Health and Environmental Control
Bureau of Health Regulations
2600 Bull Street
Columbia, SC 29201
Tel: 803-737-7202

Department of Health and Environmental Control
Bureau of Health Facilities and Services Development
2600 Bull Street
Columbia, SC 29201
Tel: 803-737-7200

HMOs

Insurance Commission
1612 Marion Street
Columbia, SC 29201
Tel: 803-737-6221

Insurance Commission
Department of Insurance
PO Box 100105
Columbus, SC 29202
Tel: 803-737-6150

South Dakota

Doctors

State Board of Medical and Osteopathic Examiners
1323 South Minnesota Avenue
Sioux Falls, SD 57105
Tel: 605-336-1965

Hospitals

Licensure and Certification Program
State Department of Health
Joe Foss Building
523 East Capitol Avenue
Pierre, SD 57501
Tel: 605-773-3364

South Dakota Department of Health
Policy & Statistics
445 East Capitol Avenue
Pierre, SD 57501-3185
Tel: 605-773-3130

HMOs

Department of Health
445 East Capitol Avenue
Pierre, SD 57501
Tel: 605-773-3361

Tennessee

Doctors

Department of Health
Health Related Boards
344 Cordell Hull Building
Nashville, TN 37247
Tel: 615-367-6220

Hospitals

Division for Licensing Health Care Facilities
283 Plus Park Boulevard
Nashville, TN 37247-0508
Tel: 615-367-6303

HMOs

Department of Health
Division of Health Care Facilities
283 Plus Park Boulevard
Nashville, TN 37247
Tel: 615-367-6316

Department of Commerce and Insurance
Policy Holders Service Section
500 James Robertson Parkway
Nashville, TN 37243
Tel: 800-342-4029

Texas

Doctors

Department of Health
State Board of Medical Examiners
1100 West 49th Street
Austin, TX 78756
Tel: 512-834-7728

Hospitals

Health Facility Licensure and Certification
Texas Department of Health
1100 West 49th Street
Austin, TX 78756
Tel: 512-834-6650

Bureau of State Health Data Policy Analysis
Texas Department of Health
1100 West 49th Street
Austin, TX 78756
Tel: 512-458-7261

Disclosure Section
Texas Department of Health
1100 West 49th Street
Austin, TX 78756
Tel: 512-834-6687

HMOs

Texas Department of Insurance
PO Box 149104
Austin, TX 78714-9104
Tel: 512-463-6500
Tel: 800-252-3439

Utah

Doctors

Business Regulation
Division of Occupational and Professional Licensing
160 East 300 South
PO Box 45805
Salt Lake City, UT 84145
Tel: 801-530-6628

Hospitals

Utah Department of Health
Bureau of Health Facility Licensure
288 North 1460 West
PO Box 16990
Salt Lake City, UT 84116-0990
Tel: 801-538-6152

HMOs

State Insurance Department
State Office Building, Suite 3110
Salt Lake City, UT 84114
Tel: 801-538-3805

Vermont

Doctors

Secretary of State Office
Board of Medical Practice
109 State Street
Montpelier, VT 05609-1106
Tel: 802-828-2673

Hospitals

Vermont Department of Health
Division of Public Health Analysis and Policy
108 Cherry Street
PO Box 70
Burlington, VT 05402
Tel: 802-863-7300

HMOs

Department of Banking, Insurance and Securities
89 Main Street, Drawer 20
Montpelier, VT 05620-3101
Tel: 802-828-3301

Virginia

Doctors

Board of Medicine
Department of Health Professions
6606 West Broad Street, 4th Floor
Richmond, VA 23230-1717
Tel: 804-662-9925

Hospitals

Office of Health Facilities Regulation
Department of Health
3600 West Broad Street, Suite 216
Richmond, VA 23230
Tel: 804-367-2102

Center for Health Statistics
PO Box 1000
Richmond, VA 23208
Tel: 804-786-6206

HMOs

State Corporation Commission
Bureau of Insurance
Box 1157
Richmond, VA 23209
Tel: 804-371-9741

Washington

Doctors

Department of Health
PO Box 47866
Olympia, WA 98504-7866
Tel: 206-753-2287

Hospitals

Department of Health
Facilities and Services Licensing
PO Box 47852
Olympia, WA 98504-7852
Tel: 206-705-6652

Department of Health
Office of Hospital Patient Data Systems
1102 South East Quince Street
PO Box 47811
Olympia, WA 98504-7811
Tel: 206-705-6003

HMOs

Office of the Insurance Commissioner
Insurance Building
PO Box 40255
Olympia, WA 98504
Tel: 206-586-0691

Office of the Insurance Commissioner
Consumer Protection
PO Box 40256
Olympia, WA 98504
Tel: 206-753-3613

West Virginia

Doctors

West Virginia Board of Medicine
101 Dee Drive
Charleston, WV 25311
Tel: 304-558-2921

Hospitals

Office of Health Facility Licensure and Certification
West Virginia Division of Health
State Capitol Complex
1900 Kanawha Boulevard E
Building 3, Room 550
Charleston, WV 25305
Tel: 304-558-0050

West Virginia Healthcare Cost Review Authority
100 Dee Drive, Suite 201
Charleston, WV 25311
Tel: 304-558-7000

HMOs

Insurance Commissioners Office
2019 Washington Street, E
Charleston, WV 23540
Tel: 304-558-3386

Wisconsin

Doctors

Wisconsin Medical Examining Board
1400 East Washington Avenue
PO Box 8935
Madison, WI 53708
Tel: 608-266-2811

Wisconsin Medical Mediation Board
110 East Main Street, Suite 320
Madison, WI 53703
Tel: 608-266-7711

Hospitals

Bureau of Quality Compliance
Department of Health & Social Services
PO Box 309
Madison, WI 53701
Tel: 608-266-8481

Office of Commissioner of Insurance
Office of Healthcare Information
121 East Wilson Street, 1st Floor
Madison, WI 53702
Tel: 608-267-0236

Record Custodian
Bureau of Quality Compliance
Division of Health
PO Box 309
Madison, WI 53701
Tel: 608-266-8481

HMOs

Office of the Commissioner of Insurance
PO Box 7873
Madison, WI 53707
Tel: 608-266-3585

Wyoming

Doctors

Wyoming Board of Medicine
Barrett Building, 2nd Floor
Cheyenne, WY 82002
Tel: 307-777-6463

Hospitals

Health Facilities Licensing Unit
Department of Health
Hathaway Building, 4th Floor
2300 Capitol Avenue
Cheyenne, WY 82002
Tel: 307-777-7123

HMOs

Wyoming Insurance Department
122 West 25th Street
Cheyenne, WY 82002
Tel: 307-777-7401

How to Use the Charts

Outlined in the following charts is commonly sought information and its availability by state.

The availability of information is denoted by the following symbols:

✓ = The information is on file and available to the public.

✕ = The information is unavailable to the public.

🖂 = The information is available but your request must be in writing.

$ = The information is available for a fee.

NH = Currently, there are no HMOs in the state.

NR = There is no state regulation. Information is available through the federal government.

DOCTORS

	Licensure	Address	Board Certification	Education / Residency	Complaints
Alabama	✓	✓	✓	✓	✓
Alaska	✓	✓	✓	✓	✓
Arizona	✓	✓	✓	✓	✓
Arkansas	✓	✓	✓	✓	✓
California	✓	✓	×	×	✓
Colorado	✓	✓	✓	✓	✓
Connecticut	✓	✓	✓	✓	✓
Delaware	✓	✓	×	✓	×
District of Col	✓	✓	×	×	✓
Florida	✓	✓	✓	✓	✉
Georgia	✓	✓	×	✓	✓
Hawaii	✓	✓	×	×	✓
Idaho	✓	✓	✓	×	✓
Illinois	✓	✓	×	✓	✓
Indiana	✓	✓	×	×	✓
Iowa	✓	✓	×	✓	✓
Kansas	✓	✓	×	✓	✓
Kentucky	✓	✓	×	✓	✓
Louisiana	✓	✓	×	✓	✓
Maine	✓	✓	✓	✓	✓
Maryland	✓	✓	×	✓	✓
Massachusetts	✓	✓	✓	×	✓
Michigan	✓	✓	×	×	✓
Minnesota	✓	✓	×	✓	×
Mississippi	✓	✓	×	×	✉
Missouri	✓	✓	×	✓	✓

Doctors

	Licensure	Address	Board Certification	Education / Residency	Complaints
Montana	✓	✓	✓	×	✓
Nebraska	✓	✓	×	×	✓
Nevada	✓	✓	✓	✓	✓
New Hamp.	✓	✓	✓	✓	✓
New Jersey	✓	✓	✓	×	✓
New Mexico	✓	✓	×	×	$
New York	✓	✓	×	×	✓
North Carol.	✓	✓	×	✓	✓
North Dakota	✓	✓	✓	✓	✓
Ohio	✓	✓	×	✓	✓
Oklahoma	✓	✓	✓	✓	✓
Oregon	✓	✓	×	✓	$
Pennsylvania	✓	✓	×	×	✓
Rhode Island	✓	✓	✓	✓	✓
South Carol.	✓	✓	✓	✓	✓
South Dakota	✓	✓	✓	✓	✓
Tennessee	✓	✓	✓	✓	✓
Texas	✓	✓	×	×	✓
Utah	✓	✓	×	✓	✓
Vermont	✓	✓	✓	✓	✓
Virginia	✓	✓	×	✓	✓
Washington	✓	✓	×	✓	✓
W Virginia	✓	✓	×	✓	✓
Wisconsin	✓	✓	×	×	✓
Wyoming	✓	✓	✓	✓	✓

HOSPITALS

	Licensure	Accreditation	Statistics	Number of Complaints	Staff Data	Directory Available
Alabama	✓	✓	✓	✗	✓	$
Alaska	✓	✓	✓	✓	✓	✓
Arizona	✓	✓	✓	✓	✓	✓
Arkansas	✓	✓	✗	✗	✗	✉
California	✓	✓	✗	✓	✗	$
Colorado	✓	✓	✗	✓	✗	✓
Connecticut	✓	✓	✓	✗	✓	✓
Delaware	✓	✓	✓	✓	✗	✓
District of Col	✓	✓	✗	✓	✗	✓
Florida	✓	✓	✓	✉	✗	✓
Georgia	✓	✓	✗	✓	✗	✓
Hawaii	✓	✓	✗	✗	✗	✓
Idaho	✓	✓	✓	✓	✗	✓
Illinois	✓	✓	✓	✗	✗	✓
Indiana	✓	✓	✗	✉	✗	✓
Iowa	✓	✓	✗	$	✗	✓
Kansas	✓	✓	✓	✓	✓	$
Kentucky	✓	✓	✓	✓	✗	✓
Louisiana	✓	✓	✗	✉	✗	$
Maine	✉	✓	✗	✓	✗	$
Maryland	✓	✓	✓	✓	✗	✓
Massachusetts	✓	✓	✓	✓	✗	✓
Michigan	✓	✓	✓	$	✗	✓
Minnesota	✓	✓	✓	✓	✓	✓
Mississippi	✓	✓	✓	✗	✗	$
Missouri	✓	✓	✗	✓	✓	$

HOSPITALS

	Licensure	Accreditation	Statistics	Number of Complaints	Staff Data	Directory Available
Montana	✓	✓	✓	✓	×	$
Nebraska	✓	✓	✓	✓	✓	✓
Nevada	✓	✓	✓	✓	×	$
New Hamp.	✓	×	✓	×	×	✓
New Jersey	✓	✓	×	✓	×	✓
New Mexico	✓	✓	✓	×	×	✓
New York	✓	×	✓	×	×	$
North Carol.	✓	✓	✓	✓	×	✓
North Dakota	✓	✓	✓	×	×	$
Ohio	✓	×	✓	×	×	$
Oklahoma	✓	✓	✓	×	×	$
Oregon	✓	✓	$	×	✓	$
Pennsylvania	✓	×	✓	×	✓	✓
Rhode Island	✓	✓	✓	✓	✓	✓
South Carol.	✓	✓	✓	✉	×	✓
South Dakota	✓	×	✓	×	✓	✓
Tennessee	✓	✓	×	✓	×	✓
Texas	✓	✓	✓	✓	×	✓
Utah	✓	✓	×	✓	×	✓
Vermont	✓	✓	✓	✓	×	✓
Virginia	✓	✓	✓	✓	×	✓
Washington	✓	✓	✓	×	×	✓
W Virginia	✓	✓	✓	✓	×	$
Wisconsin	✓	✓	$	✓	✓	✓
Wyoming	✓	✓	✓	✓	×	$

HMOs

	Licensure	Coverages / Rates	Financial	Complaints	Directory Available
Alabama	✓	×	✓	✓	✓
Alaska	NH	NH	NH	NH	NH
Arizona	✓	×	✓	✓	✓
Arkansas	✓	×	✓	✓	✓
California	✓	✓	✓	✓	$
Colorado	✓	×	✓	✓	✓
Connecticut	✓	✓	✓	✉	✓
Delaware	✓	✓	✓	✓	✓
District of Col	NH	NH	NH	NH	NH
Florida	✓	✓	✓	✓	✓
Georgia	✓	✓	✓	✓	✓
Hawaii	✓	NR	NR	NR	✓
Idaho	✓	✓	✓	✓	✓
Illinois	✓	✓	✓	✓	✓
Indiana	✓	×	✓	✓	✓
Iowa	✓	✓	✓	✓	✓
Kansas	✓	✓	✓	✓	✓
Kentucky	✓	✓	✓	✓	$
Louisiana	✓	×	✓	✓	✓
Maine	✓	×	✓	×	✓
Maryland	✓	×	✓	✓	✓
Massachusetts	✓	✓	✓	✓	✓
Michigan	✓	✓	✓	✓	✓
Minnesota	✓	✓	$	×	✓
Mississippi	✓	×	✓	✓	✓
Missouri	✓	×	✓	✓	✓

HMOs

	Licensure	Coverages / Rates	Financial	Complaints	Directory Available
Montana	✓	✓	✓	×	✓
Nebraska	✓	✓	✓	×	✓
Nevada	✓	✓	✓	✓	✓
New Hamp.	✓	✓	✓	✓	✓
New Jersey	✓	✓	✓	✓	✓
New Mexico	✓	✓	✓	✓	$
New York	✓	✓	✓	$	✓
North Carol.	✓	✓	✓	✓	✓
North Dakota	✓	✓	✓	✓	$
Ohio	✓	✓	✓	✓	✓
Oklahoma	✓	✓	✓	✓	✓
Oregon	✓	✓	✓	✓	✓
Pennsylvania	✓	✓	✓	×	✓
Rhode Island	✓	✓	✓	×	✓
South Carol.	✓	✓	✓	✓	✓
South Dakota	✓	×	✓	×	✓
Tennessee	✓	✓	✓	✓	✓
Texas	✓	✓	✓	✓	✓
Utah	✓	✓	✓	×	✓
Vermont	✓	✓	✓	✓	✓
Virginia	✓	✓	✓	✓	✓
Washington	✓	✓	✓	✓	✓
W Virginia	✓	✓	✓	✓	✓
Wisconsin	✓	✓	✓	✓	✓
Wyoming	✓	✓	✓	✓	✓

State Departments of Insurance Appendix H

Alabama	205-269-3550
Alaska	907-465-2515
Arizona	602-912-8400
Arkansas	501-686-2900
California (only from CA)	800-927-4357
Colorado	303-894-7499
Connecticut	203-297-3800
Delaware	302-577-3119
District of Columbia	202-727-8000
Florida	904-922-3131
Georgia	404-656-2056
Hawaii	808-586-2790
Idaho	208-334-2250
Illinois	217-782-4515
Indiana	317-232-2385
Iowa	515-281-5705
Kansas	913-296-3071
Kentucky	502-564-6088
Louisiana	504-342-5900
Maine	207-582-8707
Maryland	410-333-6300

Massachusetts........................617-727-7189

Michigan 517-373-0220

Minnesota...........................612-296-6319

Mississippi 601-359-3569

Missouri 314-751-4126

Montana.............................406-444-2040

Nebraska............................402-471-2201

Nevada 702-687-4270

New Hampshire.......................603-271-2661

New Jersey 609-292-5360

New Mexico..........................505-827-4500

New York...........................518-474-6600

North Carolina.......................919-733-7343

North Dakota........................701-224-2440

Ohio...............................614-644-2658

Oklahoma...........................405-521-2828

Oregon 503-378-4271

Pennsylvania.........................717-787-2317

Rhode Island 401-277-2223

South Carolina.......................803-737-6160

South Dakota........................605-773-3563

Tennessee...........................615-741-2693

Texas...............................512-322-3401

Utah 801-538-3800

Vermont 802-828-3301

Virginia.......................... 804-371-9741

Washington 206-753-7300

West Virginia..................... 304-558-3386

Wisconsin......................... 608-266-3585

Wyoming 307-777-7401

National Insurance
Consumer Helpline 1-800-942-4242

Medicare & Medicaid by State
Appendix I

Alabama

Medicaid	(205) 242-5000
Medicare	(205) 988-2244
or	(800) 292-8855

Alaska

Medicaid	(907) 465-3355
Medicare	(503) 222-6831
or	(800) 452-0125

Arizona

Medicaid	(602) 234-3655, ext. 4053
Medicare	(602) 861-1968
or	(800) 352-0411

Arkansas

Medicaid	(501) 682-8258
Medicare	(501) 378-2320
or	(800) 482-5525

California

Medicaid	(916) 657-1496
Medicare for counties of Los Angeles, Orange, San Diego, Ventura, Imperial, San Luis Obispo, Santa Barbara:	(213) 748-2311
For area codes 209, 408, 415, 510, 707, 916:	(916) 743-1583

For area codes 213, 310, 619, 714, 805, 818, 909:	(714) 435-5800
or	(800) 848-7713

Colorado

Medicaid	(303) 866-6092
Medicare	(303) 831-2661
or	(800) 332-6681

Connecticut

Medicaid	(203) 566-2934
Medicare	(203) 728-6783
(Hartford)	(203) 237-8592
(Meriden)	(800) 982-6819

Delaware

Medicaid	(302) 577-4901
Medicare	(800) 851-3535

District of Columbia

Medicaid	(202) 724-5173
Medicare	(800) 233-1124

Florida

Medicaid	(904) 488-3560
Medicare	(904) 355-8899
or	(800) 666-7586

Georgia

Medicaid	(404) 656-4479
Medicare	(912) 920-2412
or	(800) 727-0827

Hawaii

Medicaid	(808) 586-5391
Medicare	(808) 524-1240

Idaho

Medicaid	(208) 334-5795
Medicare	(208) 342-7763
or	(800) 627-2782

Illinois

Medicaid	(217) 782-2570
Medicare	(312) 938-8000
or	(800) 642-6930

Indiana

Medicaid	(317) 233-4455
Medicare	(317) 842-4151
or	(800) 622-4792

Iowa

Medicaid	(515) 281-8794
Medicare	(515) 245-4785
or	(800) 532-1285

Kansas

Medicaid	(913) 296-3981
Medicare for counties of Johnson and Wyandotte:	(816) 561-0900
or	(800) 892-5900
for rest of state:	(913) 232-3773
or	(800) 432-3531

Kentucky

Medicaid	(502) 564-4321
Medicare	(502) 425-6759
or	(800) 999-7608

Louisiana

Medicaid	(504) 342-3891
Medicare	(800) 462-9666
in New Orleans:	(504) 529-1494
in Baton Rouge:	(504) 927-3490

Maine

Medicaid	(207) 287-2674
Medicare	(207) 828-4300
or	(800) 492-0919

Maryland

Medicaid	(410) 225-6505
Medicare	(410) 561-4160
or	(800) 492-4795

Massassachusetts

Medicaid	(617) 348-5691
Medicare	(617) 741-3300
or	(800) 882-1228

Michigan

Medicaid	(517) 335-5001
Medicare	(313) 225-8200
or	(800) 482-4045

Minnesota

Medicaid	(612) 296-8818
Medicare for counties of	
Anoka, Dakota, Fillmore:	(612) 884-7171
or	(800) 352-2762
for rest of state:	(612) 456-5070
or	(800) 392-0343

Mississippi

Medicaid	(601) 359-6050
Medicare	(601) 956-0372
or	(800) 682-5417

Missouri

Medicaid	(314) 751-3425
Medicare for counties of Andrew, Atchison, Bates, Benton, Buchannon, Caldwell, Carroll, Cass, Clay, Clinton, Daviess, DeKalb, Gentry, Grundy, Harrison, Henry, Holt, Jackson, Johnson, LaFayette, Livingston, Mercer, Nodaway, Pettis, Platte, Ray, St. Clair, Saline, Vernon and Worth:	(816) 561-0900
or	(800) 892-5900
for rest of state:	(314) 843-8880
or	(800) 392-3070

Montana

Medicaid	(406) 444-4540
Medicare	(406) 444-8350

Nebraska

Medicaid	(402) 471-9718
Medicare	(913) 232-3773

Nevada

Medicaid	(702) 687-4378
Medicare	(602) 861-1968
or	(800) 528-0311

New Hampshire

Medicaid	(603) 271-4353
Medicare	(207) 828-4300
or	(800) 447-1142

New Jersey

Medicaid	(609) 588-2600
Medicare	(717) 975-7333
or	(800) 462-9306

New Mexico

Medicaid	(505) 827-4315
Medicare	(505) 821-3350
or	(800) 423-2925

New York

Medicaid	(518) 474-9132
Medicare for counties of Bronx, Columbia, Delaware, Dutchess, Greene, Kings, Nassau, New York, Orange, Putnam, Richmond, Rockland, Suffolk, Sullivan, Ulster, Westchester:	(516) 244-5100
or	(800) 442-8430

for county of Queens:	(212) 721-1770
for rest of state:	(607) 772-6906
or	(800) 252-6550

North Carolina

Medicaid	(919) 733-2060
Medicare	(919) 665-0348
or	(800) 672-3071

North Dakota

Medicaid	(701) 224-2321
Medicare	(701) 282- 0691
or	(800) 247-2267

Ohio

Medicaid	(614) 644-0140
Medicare	(614) 249-7157
or	(800) 282-0530

Oklahoma

Medicaid	(405) 525-1091
Medicare	(405) 848-7711
or	(800) 522-9079

Oregon

Medicaid	(503) 378-2263
Medicare	(503) 222-6831
or	(800) 452-0125

Pennsylvania

Medicaid	(717) 787-1870
Medicare	(717) 763-3601
or	(800) 382-1274

Rhode Island

Medicaid	(401) 464-3575
Medicare	(401) 861-2273
or	(800) 662-5170

South Carolina

Medicaid	(803) 253-6100
Medicare	(803) 788-3882
or	(800) 868-2522

South Dakota

Medicaid	(605) 773-3495
Medicare	(701) 282-0691
or	(800) 437-4762

Tennessee

Medicaid	(615) 741-0213
Medicare	(615) 244-5650
or	(800) 342-8900

Texas

Medicaid	(512) 450-3050
Medicare	(214) 235-3433
or	(800) 442-2620

Utah

Medicaid	(801) 538-6111
Medicare	(801) 481-6196
or	(800) 426-3477

Vermont

Medicaid	(802) 241-2880
Medicare	(207) 828-4300
or	(800) 447-1142

Virginia

Medicaid	(804) 786-7933
Medicare for cities of Alexandria, Falls Church, Fairfax:	(717) 763-3601
or	(800) 233-1124
for rest of state:	(804) 330-4786
or	(800) 552-3423

Washington

Medicaid	(206) 753-1777
Medicare	(206) 621-0359
or	(800) 372-6604

West Virginia

Medicaid	(304) 926-1700
Medicare	(614) 249-7157
or	(800) 848-0106

Wisconsin

Medicaid	(608) 266-2522
Medicare	(608) 221-3330
or	(800) 944-0051

Wyoming

Medicaid	(307) 777-7531
Medicare	(307) 632-9381
or	(800) 442-2371

Medigap Plans
Appendix J

Plan A

Plan A, which must be offered by every insurer, is the basic Medigap plan and provides certain core benefits. These are:

1. Coverage for Part A coinsurance—the daily amount you must pay for hospitalization if you are hospitalized from 61 to 90 days. The coinsurance in 1994 was $174 per day.
2. Coverage for Part A coinsurance for a hospital stay extending from 91 to 150 days. In 1994, this amount was $48 per day.
3. Coverage for an extra 365 days of hospitalization after you have exhausted all of your Medicare benefits.
4. Coverage of the Part A blood deductible: the cost of the first three pints of blood you may need as an inpatient in a hospital.
5. Coverage for Part B coinsurance: 20 percent of Medicare's allowable charge.

Plan B

1. Core benefits as listed in Plan A.
2. Coverage for coinsurance for a stay in a skilled care nursing facility lasting from 21 to 100 days. In 1994, this amount was $87 daily.
3. Part A hospital deductible was $696 per benefit period in 1994.

Plan C

1. Core benefits.
2. Coverage for coinsurance for a stay in a skilled nursing facility.
3. Part A hospital deductible.
4. Emergency medical care in foreign countries.
5. Part B deductible, $100 per calendar year. After that, Medicare picked up 80 percent of the cost in 1994.

Plan D

1. Core benefits.
2. Coverage of coinsurance for a stay in a skilled nursing facility.
3. Part A hospital deductible.
4. Emergency medical care in foreign countries.
5. Short-term coverage for home care following an injury, illness, or surgery. This benefit is limited to $1,600 per year and covers assistance with activities of daily living such as eating, bathing, and dressing. Care must be provided by a licensed home-health aide, homemaker, or personal care worker.

Plan E

1. Core benefits.
2. Coverage for coinsurance for a stay in a skilled nursing facility.
3. Part A hospital deductible.
4. Emergency medical care in foreign countries.
5. Preventive medical care, including the cost of annual physical examinations, fecal occult blood tests, mammograms, thyroid and diabetes screening, a pure-tone hearing test, and cholesterol screening every five years.

Plan F

1. Core benefits.
2. Coverage for coinsurance for a stay in a skilled nursing facility.
3. Part A hospital deductibles.
4. Part B deductible.
5. Emergency medical care in foreign countries.
6. 100 percent of Medicare Part B excess charges, the difference between Medicare's allowed charge and the amount the physician actually bills.

Plan G

1. Core benefits.
2. Coverage for coinsurance for a stay in a skilled nursing facility.
3. Part A hospital deductible.
4. Emergency medical care in foreign countries.
5. Coverage for home care following an injury, illness, or surgery.
6. 80 percent of Medicare Part B excess charges.

Plan H

1. Core benefits.
2. Coverage for coinsurance for a stay in a skilled nursing facility.
3. Emergency medical care in foreign countries.
4. Coverage for home care following an injury, illness, or surgery.
5. 50 percent of the cost of prescription drugs up to a maximum annual benefit of $1,250. The policyholder must first satisfy a $250 annual deductible.

Plan I

1. Core benefits.
2. Part A hospital deductible.
3. Emergency medical care in foreign countries.
4. Coverage for home care following an injury, illness, or surgery.
5. 100 percent of Part B excess charges.
6. The basic prescription drug benefit (See Plan H).

Plan J

1. Core benefits.
2. Coverage for coinsurance for a stay in a skilled nursing facility.
3. Part A hospital deductible.
4. Part B hospital deductible.
5. Emergency medical care in foreign countries.
6. Coverage for home care following an injury, illness, or surgery.
7. Preventive medical care.
8. 100 percent of Part B excess charges.
9. 50 percent of the cost of prescription drugs up to an annual maximum benefit of $3,000 after a $250 annual deductible has been met.

Certified Regional Poison Control Centers Appendix K

This handy reference list of emergency numbers to call in case of accidental poisoning should be placed in a convenient place so that anyone in your family can find it quickly, if necessary. If someone swallows a substance believed to be poison, phone the nearest poison control center which is staffed with physicians, pharmacologists, pharmacists, and registered nurses. These medical professionals will give you information about antidotes and appropriate first aid care.

The centers practice prevention as well as deal with acute problems. Consumers may call for general information and literature.

All of the centers listed here are certified by the American Association for Poison Control Centers.

Verify the number(s) for your region on a regular basis to ensure accuracy.

Alabama

Regional Poison Control Center

The Children's Hospital of Alabama
1600 7th Avenue South
Birmingham, AL 35233-1711

Emergency	(205) 939-9201
(AL only)	(800) 292-6678
or	(205) 933-4050

Arizona

Arizona Poison and Drug Information Center

Arizona Health Sciences Center, Room #3204-K
1501 N Campbell Avenue
Tucson, AZ 85724

Emergency	(602) 626-6016
(AZ only)	(800) 362-0101

Samaritan Regional Poison Center

1441 North 12th Street
1130 E McDowell, Suite A-5
Phoenix, AZ 85006
Emergency (602) 253-3334

California

Fresno Regional Poison Control Center of Fresno Community Hospital and Medical Center

3151 North Millbrook
Fresno, CA 93703
Emergency (800) 346-5922
or (209) 445-1222

San Diego Regional Poison Center

UCSD Medical Center; 8925
200 West Arbor Drive Box 8925
San Diego, CA 92103-8925
Emergency (619) 543-6000
(619 area code) (800) 876-4766

San Francisco Bay Area Regional Poison Control Center

San Francisco General Hospital
1001 Potrero Avenue, Building 80, Room 230
San Francisco, CA 94122
Emergency (800) 523-2222

Santa Clara Valley Medical Center Regional Poison Center

750 South Bascom Avenue
San Jose, CA 95128
Emergency (408) 299-5112
(CA only) (800) 662-9886

University of California, Davis, Medical Center Regional Poison Center

Control Center
2315 Stockton Boulevard
Sacramento, CA 95817
Emergency (916) 734-3692
(Northern CA only) (800) 342-9293

LA Regional Drug and Poison Information Center

1200 North State Street
Los Angelos, CA 90033

Emergency	(800) 777-6476
	(213) 222-3212
(Southern CA only)	(800) 544-4404

Colorado

Rocky Mountain Poison Center

645 Bannock Street
Denver, CO 80204

Emergency	(303) 629-1123

District of Columbia

National Capital Poison Center

3201 New Mexico Avenue NW
Washington, DC 20016

Emergency	(202) 625-3333

Florida

The Florida Poison Information Center at Tampa General Hospital

Post Office Box 1289
Tampa, FL 33606

Emergency	(800) 282-3171
(in Tampa)	(813) 253-4444

Georgia

Georgia Poison Center

Grady Memorial Hospital
80 Butler Street SE
Atlanta, GA 30335-3801

Emergency	(800) 282-5846
(GA only)	(404) 616-9000

Indiana

Indiana Poison Center

Methodist Hospital of Indiana
21st and I-65
PO Box 1367
Indianapolis, IN 46206-1367

Emergency	(800) 382-9097
(IN only)	(317) 929-2323

Kentucky

Kentucky Regional Poison Center of Kosair Children's Hospital

PO Box 35070
Louisville, KY 40232-5070

Emergency	(800) 722-5725
(KY only)	(502) 629-7275

Maryland

Maryland Poison Center

20 N. Pine Street
Baltimore, MD 21201

Emergency	(410) 528-7701
(MD only)	(800) 492-2414

National Capital Poison Center (DC suburbs only)

3201 New Mexico Ave. NW
Washington, DC 20016

Emergency	(202) 625-3333

Massachusetts

Massachusetts Poison Control Center

300 Longwood Avenue
Boston, MA 02115

Emergency	(617) 232-2120
or	(800) 682-9211

Michigan

Blodgett Regional Poison Center

1840 Wealthy SE
Grand Rapids, MI 49506-2968

Emergency (MI only)	(800) 632-2727
TTY	(800) 356-3232

Poison Control Center

Children's Hospital of Michigan - Poison Control Center
3901 Beaubien Boulevard
Detroit, MI 48201

Emergency	(313) 745-5711
	(800)-POISON-1

Minnesota

Hennepin Regional Poison Center

Hennepin County Medical Center
701 Park Avenue
Minneapolis, MN 55415

Emergency	(612) 347-3141
Petline	(612) 337-7387
TDD	(612) 337-7474

Minnesota Regional Poison Center

640 Jackson Street
St. Paul, MN 55101

Emergency	(612) 221-2113

Missouri

Cardinal Glennon Children's Hospital Regional Poison Center

1465 S Grand Boulevard
St. Louis, MO 63104

Emergency	(314) 772-5200
or	(800) 366-8888

Montana

Rocky Mountain Poison Center

645 Bannock Street
Denver, CO 80204
Emergency (303) 629-1123

Nebraska

The Poison Center

8301 Dodge Street
Omaha, NE 68114
Emergency (800) 955-9119
(in Omaha) (402) 390-5555

New Jersey

New Jersey Poison Information and Education System

201 Lyons Avenue
Newark, NJ 07112
Emergency (800) 962-1253
(800) POISON-1

New Mexico

New Mexico Poison and Drug Information Center

University of New Mexico
Albuquerque, NM 87131-1076
Emergency (505) 843-2551
(NM only) (800) 432-6866

New York

Long Island Regional Poison Control Center

Winthrope University Hospital
259 First Street
Mineola, NY 11501
Emergency (516) 542-2323, 2324

New York City Poison Control Center

NYC Department of Health
455 First Avenue, Room 123
New York, NY 10016

Emergency	(212) 340-4494
or	(212) P-O-I-S-O-N-S
TDD	(212) 689-9014

Ohio

Central Ohio Poison Center

700 Children's Drive
Columbus, OH 43205-2696

Emergency	(614) 228-1323
or	(800) 682-7625
TTY	(614) 228-2272
or	(614) 722-2636

Cincinnati Drug & Poison Information Center and Regional Poison Control System

P.O. Box 670144
Cincinnati, OH 45267-0144

Emergency	(513) 558-5111
(OH only)	(800) 872-5111

Oregon

Oregon Poison Center

Oregon Health Sciences University
3181 SW Sam Jackson Park Road
Portland, OR 97201

Emergency	(503) 494-8968
(OR only)	(800) 452-7165

Pennsylvania

Central Pennsylvania Poison Center

University Hospital
Milton S Hershey Medical Center
Hershey, PA 17033

Emergency	(717) 531-6111

The Poison Control (serving the greater Philadelphia metropolitan area)

One Children's Center
Philadelphia, PA 19104-4303
Emergency (215) 386-2100
(800) 722-7112

Pittsburgh Poison Center

3705 Fifth Avenue @ DeSoto Street
Pittsburgh, PA 15213
Emergency (412) 681-6669

Texas

North Texas Poison Center

PO Box 35926
Dallas, TX 75235
Emergency (214) 590-5000
Texas Watts (800) 441-0040

Utah

The Utah Poison Control Center

410 Chipeta Way, Ste. 230
Salt Lake City, UT 84108
Emergency (801) 581-2151
(UT only) (800) 456-7707

Virginia

Blue Ridge Poison Center

Box 67
Blue Ridge Hospital
Charlottesville, VA 22901
Emergency (800) 451-1428

West Virginia

West Virginia Poison Center

3110 MacCorkle Avenue, SE
Charleston, WV 25304

Emergency	(800) 642-3625
(WV only)	(304) 348-4211

Wyoming

The Poison Center

8301 Dodge Street
Omaha, NE 68114

Emergency (Omaha)	(402) 390-5555
(NE)	(800) 955-9119

Help Lines & Numbers of Interest Appendix L

The following listings describe help and information lines offered by various organizations covering information on a wide variety of health problems and issues. Many are toll-free numbers. They are organized alphabetically by topic.

Accreditation

Joint Commission on Accreditation of Healthcare Organizations

Information available regarding the accreditation status of health care providers, especially hospitals

1 Renaissance Boulevard
Oak Brook Terrace, IL 60181
708-916-5600

National Committee for Quality Assurance

Information available on accreditation of HMOs and other managed care organizations

1350 New York Avenue, Suite 700
Washington, DC 20005
202-628-5788

American Association of Homes for the Aging

Offers information on accreditation status of homes and free listings of AAHA accredited homes

901 E Street NW
Washington, DC 20004
202-783-2242

American Health Care Association

Information available on institutional long term care facilities and nursing homes

1201 L Street N.W
Washington, DC 20005
202-842-4444

National Consumers League

Information on Food and Drug Administration and health care reforms

815 15th Street NW, Suite 928
Washington, DC 20005
202-639-8140
800-876-7060 (National fraud information center)

Adoption

Adopt a Special Kid (AASK) America

Offers information on how to adopt a child

510-451-1748

Edna Gladney Center

Adoption agency/maternity home offering legal assistance, counseling, etc.

2300 Hemphill
Fort Worth, TX 76110
800-433-2922

National Adoption Center

Clearinghouse for information relating to adoption—matches children with prospective adoptive parent(s)

800-TO-ADOPT

AIDS

Aids Clinical Information Service

Library and referrals available to assist people in getting into clinical studies and trials

PO Box 6421
Rockville, MD 20849-6421
800-874-2572
800-243-7012 (TTY–TDD)
301-217-0032 (International Number)

American Indian Community House: HIV/AIDS Project

Offers alcoholism rehabilitation/counseling, legal services, job training and support groups

404 Lafayette Street, 2nd Floor
New York, NY 10003
212-598-0100

American Red Cross National Headquarters AIDS Education

Educational programs, AIDS one-on-one courses, referrals and blood tests available

17th and D Streets, NW
Washington, DC 20006
202-434-4074

Asian and Pacific Islander Coalition on HIV/AIDS (APICHA)

Offers multilingual prevention education programs, counseling and support groups

41 John Street, 3rd Floor
New York, NY 10038
212-349-3293

Body Positive

Information, referrals and support groups for HIV+ individuals, lovers and spouses

2095 Broadway
Suite 306
New York, NY 10023
212-721-1346

Centers For Disease Control and Prevention National AIDS Clearinghouse

Answer AIDS questions, send out informational material: statistics, referrals, etc.

PO Box 6003
Rockville, MD 20849-6003
800-458-5231
800-342-AIDS (English Hotline)
800-344-SIDA (Spanish Hotline)
800-243-7012 (TT)
301-738-6616 (fax)

Clinical Partners

AIDS care, counseling and education

800-483-8883

Gay Men's Health Crisis Line

Educational programs, publications, legal services and HIV+ client support groups, counseling and recreation services

212-807-6655

National Association of People with AIDS

Provides information and referrals to local chapters of People With AIDS

2025 I Street, NW Suite 1118
Washington, DC 20006
202-898-0414

National Leadership Coalition on AIDS

National membership organization focusing on workplace policies and issues

1730 M Street NW, Suite 905
Washington, DC 20036
202-429-0930

National Native American AIDS Prevention Center

Free information available including referrals to testing and counseling centers

3515 Grand Avenue, Suite 100
Oakland, CA 94610
800-283-2437
510-444-2051 (Oakland)

Project Inform

Information available on treatment options, referrals, outreach and advocacy programs

800-822-7422
800-334-7422 – California only

Teens Teaching AIDS and Prevention

Answers questions about AIDS and/or AIDS related topics, will send free literature

800-234-8336 (4:00–8:00 PM CST)

Air Quality

National Indoor Air Quality Information Clearinghouse

Distribution of literature on air quality

PO Box 37133
Washington, DC 20013
800-438-4318
202-484-1307
202-484-1510 (fax)

Allergies/Asthma

Allergy Information Referral Line
American Academy of Allergy and Immunology Hotline

Sends out informational pamphlets and serves as an allergist referral service

800-822-ASMA

American College of Allergy and Immunology

Information available on treatments available to allergy sufferers

800-842 7777

Asthma and Allergy Foundation of America

Educational literature available as well as maps depicting plant-growth zones known to cause allergies

1717 Massachusetts Avenue, NW, Suite 105
Washington, DC 10026
800-727-8462
202-466-7643 – District of Columbia only

National Institute of Allergy and Infectious Diseases Office of Communications

Distributes information to the public on allergies and infectious diseases

Building 31, Room 7A50
9000 Rockville Pike
Bethesda, MD 20892
301-496-5717 (8:30 AM–5:00 PM EST, M–F)
301-402-0120 (fax)

National Jewish Asthma Center

Answers questions, has information available about allergies, asthma and related topics and will refer out to local allergists

1400 Jackson Street
Denver, CO 80206
800-222-5864

Alternative Medicine

American Massage Therapy Association

Literature and referrals available

1130 West North Shore Avenue
Chicago, IL 60626
312-761-2682

American Society of Clinical Hypnosis

Literature and referrals available

708-297-3317

Integral Yoga Institute

Information and referrals available

227 West 13th Street
New York, NY 10011
212-929-0585

Office of Alternative Medicine (OAM)

Facilitates the evaluation of alternative medical treatment modalities to help determine their effectiveness and bring alternative medicine in to mainstream medicine. This agency does not provide referrals but they are in the process of setting up a clearinghouse of information

Bethesda, MD
301-402-2466

Traditional Acupuncture Institute

Clinic offering information and referrals on acupuncture.

American City Building, Suite 108
Columbia, MD 21044
301-596-3675

Alzheimer's Disease

The Alzheimer's Association

(8:30 AM–5:00 PM EST)
800-272-3900 – Toll free information and referral service

Alzheimer's Disease Education and Referral Center

Offers information and literature on Alzheimer's Disease and refers out to physicians and/or other organizations when necessary

PO Box 8250
Silver Spring, MD 20907
800-438-4380 (8:30 AM–5:00 PM EST)
301-587-4352 (fax)

The Helmsley Alzheimer Alert Program

Patient "wanderers program" (ID bracelet and emergency number), family counseling, and home services

800-733-9596

Anemia

Cooley's Anemia Foundation

Supports research, offers literature and support groups

129-09 26th Avenue
Flushing, NY 11354
800-522-7222
718-321-2873

National Association for Sickle Cell Disease

Offers educational and training programs and materials to the public and provides diagnostic screening

800-421-8453
213-736-5455 – Los Angeles only

Arthritis

Arthritis Foundation Information Line

Informational literature available on arthritis and related problems

800-283-7800
212-477-8310 (New York Chapter)

National Arthritis Foundation Information Line Information Clearinghouse

Information specialists available to answer questions and send out free publications

PO Box AMS
9000 Rockville Pike
Bethesda, MD 20892
301-495-4484
301-587-4352 (fax)

Autism

Autism Society of America

Information and referral service

7910 Woodmont Avenue, Suite 650
Bethesda, MD 20814-3015
301-565-0433 (9:00 AM–5:00 PM EST)

Birth Defects

The March of Dimes

Prevention of birth defects—funding of prenatal and drug treatment programs, educational campaigns, AIDS education, funds research into birth defects; local chapters in each county

233 Park Avenue South
New York, NY 10003
212-353-8353

Spina Bifida Association of America

Spina Bifida information and referral

800-621-3141
202-944-3285 – Washington, DC only

Blindness

American Council of the Blind

Recorded messages updated periodically outlining information on events of interest to the blind

202-331-1058 ACB electronic bulletin board
800-424-8666 (6:00 PM–Midnight)
202-467-5081

American Foundation for the Blind Hotline

Answers questions, operates a referral service, offers literature on consumer products, catalogs for videos, publications, etc.

800-232-5463
202-457-1487 (Eastern Regional Office
Washington, DC)

Blind Children's Center

Infant stimulation programs, parent participation groups, preschools, family support services, research programs, interdisciplinary programs and publication of braille books

800-222-3566

National Society to Prevent Blindness

Educational/informational hotline with free literature available, professional public information

800-221-3004

National Library Service for the Blind and Physically Handicapped

Books available for borrow or rent in large print and/or braille

Library of Congress
1291 Taylor Street NW
Washington, DC 20542
800-424-8567
202-707-5100
202-707-0712 (fax)

Recording for the Blind

Recordings of literature available

800-221-4792

Boating Safety

Office of Navigation Safety and Waterway Services

Information available about boating/Coast Guard law and regulations and safety of waterways

US Coast Guard Auxiliary; Auxiliary Boating and Consumer Affairs Division (G–NAB)
2100 Second Street SW
Washington, DC 20593-0001
800-368-5647 (Boating Safety Hotline)
202-267-0780 – in Metropolitan Washington, DC only

Breast Cancer

Breast Cancer Hotline
Physicians Committee for Responsible Medicine

800-875-4837

The Y-Me National Organization for Breast Cancer Information and Support

National support hotline answered by breast cancer survivors to answer questions on breast cancer

800-221-2141

Cancer

The AMC Cancer Information Center
American Medical Center Cancer Research Center

Information and counseling services

800-525-3777 (8:30 AM–5:00 PM MST)
303-233-6501

American Cancer Society

Education: screenings for skin cancer, Great American Smokeout, breast cancer awareness; patient services (local) and research—brochures and other information available; refer to local chapters

1599 Clifton Road, NE
Atlanta, GA 30329
800-ACS-2345
212-586-8700 (New York City Chapter)
404-320-3333 – Atlanta only

American Institute for Cancer Research Nutrition Hotline

Information on diet and nutrition in cancer prevention and how diet can be used in cancer treatment

1759 R Street, NW
Washington, DC 20009
800-843-8114

American International Hospital Cancer Program

Information about programs and facilities for cancer treatment available

Zion, IL
800-FOR-HELP
800-955-2822 (Customer Service)

Cancer Information Center

Offers information and answers questions about cancer and related problems

Building 31, Room 10A16
9000 Rockville Pike
Bethesda, MD 20892
800-4-CANCER

Cancer Memorial Donations-American Institute for Cancer Research

Researches on how to lower incidence of cancer through nutrition and education; literature available

800-843-8114

Leukemia Society of America

Literature available on patient aid, bone marrow transplants, melanoma, childhood leukemia, family support groups

800-955-4LSA
212-573-8484 (National Headquarters)

National Alliance for Breast Cancer Organization (NABCO)

Information and referral line

1180 Avenue of the Americas
New York, NY 10036
212-719-0154
212-719-0394 in emergencies

National Cancer Institute
Cancer Information Service NIH/Office of Cancer Communications

Cancer information and referral line which also maintains a list of American College of Radiology certified mammography programs

Building 31, Room 10A24
9000 Rockville Pike
Bethesda, MD 20892
800-4-CANCER

Cerebral Palsy

United Cerebral Palsy Association

Provides support and information on Cerebral Palsy and refers out to local chapters

800-872-5827
212-947-5770 (New York State Office)

Child Abuse

Child Help USA, Child Abuse Hot Line

Emergency services for children as well as providing literature, book lists and national statistics

800-422-4453

National Clearinghouse on Child Abuse and Neglect and Family Violence Information

Offers information on abuse, neglect and related topics

PO Box 1182
Washington, DC 20013
800-FYI-3366
703-385-7565
703-385-3206 (fax)

National Council on Child Abuse

A twenty-four hour crisis hotline operated with trained therapists available

800-222-2000 (referrals only)
800-422-4453

Children & Teens

Association for the Care of Children's Health

Educational and advocacy organization promoting family-centered care to promote quality, comprehensive health care in hospitals and other health care settings

3615 Wisconsin Avenue, NW
Washington, DC 20016
301-654-6549

Child Care Information Service

Provides information on and a referral service for accredited child care programs across the nation

Washington, DC
800-424-2460

Child Find

Assists in search for missing children (up to 18 years of age) and assist in search for abducted children

800-IAM-LOST (426-5678)

Children's Hospice International

Lends medical, psychological, emotional and spiritual support to terminally ill children and their families to enable them to live their lives to their fullest potential

800-24-CHILD

Children's Wish Foundation

Grants wishes to terminally ill children

800-323-9474

Covenant House

Runaway and youth crisis hotline to assist them in returning home and/or finding intermediary shelter

800-999-9999

Growing Up Healthy

Information available on adolescent care, prenatal care, child health concerns

New York State Department of Health
8th Floor, Room 821
Empire State Plaza
Albany, NY 12237
800-522-5006

Kevin Collins Foundation for Missing Children

Helps locate missing children by printing flyers and abduction prevention guides

800-272-0012

Missing Children Help Center

Helps locate missing children by exposing posters and prints nationwide

800-872-5437

National Association for the Education of the Young

Referrals available to accredited child care programs

800-424-2460

National Center (Hotline) for Missing and Exploited Children

Clearinghouse of information providing technical assistance to police to assist families in locating missing children

800-843-5678

National Child Watch Campaign

Information available on child safety and kidnapping prevention, and counseling available for parents of kidnapped or missing children

800-222-1464

National Clearinghouse on Child Abuse and Neglect And Family Violence Information

Collects and distributes information: topical bibliographies available, referrals, hot line numbers

PO Box 1182
Washington, DC 20013
800-FYI-3366
703-385-7565
703-385-3206 (fax)

National Clearinghouse on Family Support and Children's Mental Health

Information and literature available on subjects regarding family and childhood mental health

800-628-1696

National Information Center for Children and Youth with Disabilities

Clearinghouse of information regarding education of children with disabilities and other general information to parents

PO Box 1492
Washington, DC 20013
800-695-0285
202-884-8200
202-884-8441 (fax)

National Runaway Hotline Office of the Governor

Provides assistance to children and teens who have run away from home by referring to shelters and getting messages to families

800-392-3352 – Texas only

National Runaway Switchboard

Crisis intervention hotline for runaway or homeless youth and their families

800-621-4000

National Sudden Infant Death Syndrome Resource Center

Maintains a data base to answer questions or do searches on specific topics relating to SIDS. Also maintains a referral service for counseling, research, etc.

8201 Greensboro Drive, Suite 600
McLean, VA 22102
703-821-8955
703-821-2098 (fax)

Runaway Hotline

Provides information to runaways on shelter, counseling, medical services, etc.

800-231-6946
800-392-3352 – Texas only

Toughlove International

Forms support groups for parents of children with behavioral problems

800-333-1069

Vanished Children's Alliance

National missing childrens service which provides education in schools, distributes posters, fingerprints children and provides support groups for parents for any type of abductions, etc.

800-VANISHED (826-4743)

Youth Crisis Hotline

Provides twenty-four hour call-in counseling for children and teens, searches for lost or abducted children and advocates for abused children

800-442-4673

Youth Force (Citizen's Committee)

Community organizing, peer counseling, and youth empowerment training—literature available

305 7th Avenue, 7th Floor
New York, NY 10001
212-989-0909

Youth With Disabilities

Provides information on programs open to handicapped youths

800-333-6293

Choice In Dying

Choice In Dying

Provides counseling on choices and information on living wills

200 Varick Street
New York, NY 10014
212-366-5540
800-989-WILL

Chronic Disease

Center for Chronic Disease and Prevention

Health promotion and education database, cancer and AIDS prevention and control database

404-488-5401
404-488-5971

Cleft Palate

Cleft Palate Foundation

Refers people to physicians and support groups and offers general information

800-24-CLEFT

Consumer Services

Consumer Information & Product Safety Consumer Information Center

Clearinghouse for government consumer information available through a catalogue containing over two hundred publications on a variety of subjects

General Services Administration
Room G142
18th and F Streets NW
Washington, DC 20405
202-501-1794
202-501-4281 (fax)

Consumer Product Safety Commission Hotline

Information on unsafe consumer products

5401 Westbard Avenue, Room 332
Bethesda, MD 20207
800-638-2772
800-638-8270 (TT)
800-492-8104 (TT) – Maryland only
301-504-0580
301-504-0046 (fax)

National Consumers League

Familiar with consumer issues in health care, this agency publishes a newsletter every three months

815 15th Street NW, Suite 928
Washington, DC 20005
202-639-8140

Cystic Fibrosis

The Cystic Fibrosis Foundation

Clearinghouse of information for patients with CF, also provides a discount pharmacy and home health care. Specific Care Centers in different states

800-FIGHT-CF

Deafness And Hearing Impairments

American Speech Language Hearing Association, Hearing & Speech Helpline

General information packet and referrals to appropriate organizations are available

800-638-8255
301-897-8682 – Maryland only

Better Hearing Institute

Clearinghouse of information on hearing loss

800-327-9355
703-642-0580

Captioned Films and Videos for the Deaf
(US Department Of Education)

Free captioned film and video loan service (Must have one hearing impaired person per household)

800-237-6213

Deafness Research Foundation

Raises research money for finding the causes, treatments and prevention of deafness

800-535-3323

Hearing Aid Helpline

Provides information on hearing loss and hearing aids and referrals to hearing specialists

20361 Middlebelt
Livonia, MI 48152
800-521-5247

The Hearing Helpline, Better Hearing Institute

Provides educational materials on hearing and hearing loss

800-EARWELL

Hearing and Screening Test

Provides phone numbers in your area where you may obtain a hearing screening test

800-222-EARS

National Institute in Deafness and Other Communication Disorders Information Clearinghouse

Clearinghouse of information on deafness and other communication disorders

1 Communication Avenue
Bethesda, Maryland
20892-3456
301-907-8830 (fax)

Tripod Grapevine

Information and referral service for parents of deaf or hard of hearing children

800-352-8888

Dentistry

American Association of Oral and Maxillofacial Surgeons

Makes referrals and provides information on oral surgeons

800-822-6637

American Dental Association

General information available through consultants, free literature and referrals

211 East Chicago Avenue
Chicago, IL 60611
312-440-2500

Diabetes

American Diabetes Association

Clearinghouse for publications on diabetes, newsletter and information on public meetings

800-232-3472

American Association of Diabetes Educators

Multi-disciplinary organization of Continuing Education and Certificate Programs for Medical Professionals involved with the treatment of diabetes

800-338-3633

Diabetes Center, Inc.

Mail order service for diabetic supplies including a pharmacy

800-888-1132

The Juvenile Diabetes Foundation International

Fund raising organization for diabetes research

800-JDF-CURE

National Diabetes Information Clearinghouse

Information available on diabetes; provides literature searches for specific topics; diabetes specialist on staff to answer any specific questions

301-654-3327
301-496-2830 (fax)

Digestive Disorders

Chron's & Colitis Foundation

Raises funds for research into the causes and cure of chron's disease and colitis; provides patient education and support as well as physician education

800-932-2423
212-685-3440

National Digestive Diseases Information Clearinghouse

Information on digestive diseases and literature searches are available for specific topics; information specialist on staff to answer any specific questions

301-654-3810
301-907-8906 (fax)

Disabilities

Clearinghouse on Disability Information

Office of Special Education and Rehabilitative Services Department of Education

OSERS/Department of Education
330 C Street SW Room 3132
Washington, DC 20202
202-205-5465

Health Resource Center for People With Disabilities

Information clearinghouse on post-secondary (after high school) education opportunities for people with disabilities

800-544-3284

Disease Control

Centers for Disease Control

Federal agency which monitors and regulates health and quality of life by the prevention of disease, injury and disability

Public Inquiries
1600 Clifton Road, NE
Atlanta, GA 30333
404-639-3534

Divorce

Divorce Support

Group support for separated, divorced or people with marital problems, with a focus on recovery

312-286-4541

North American Conference of Separated & Divorced Catholics

401-943-7903

Down's Syndrome

National Down's Syndrome Congress

An advocate for people with Down's Syndrome, providing accurate and up to date information on Down's, as well as local parent group networks in every state

800-232-6372

National Down's Syndrome Society

Provides information to parents and physicians on Down's Syndrome

800-221-4602
212-460-9330

Dyslexia

The Orton Dyslexia Society

Refers to appropriate sources for testing and remediation, parent workshops, teacher training, adult support groups

800-ABCD-123
212-691-1930 – New York branch

Eating Disorders

Anorexia/Bulimia
The American Anorexia/Bulimia Association

Supply information, referrals, support groups, educational programs and professional training for social workers, psychologists and psychiatrists treating eating disorders

212-891-8686

Florida Institute of Technology-Addiction Hotline (FIT-AHL)

Literature available, overeaters anonymous referrals, counselors available to discuss treatment options

800-872-0088

Elderly Care

Alcohol Rehabilitation for the Elderly

Treatment center, referrals and information available

800-354-7089
800-344-0824

American Association of Retired Persons (AARP)

A membership organization for people fifty years and older which offers services such as: discounts on health, homeowners and automobile insurance, discounts on car rentals and hotels; an investment program; a monthly bulletin and a magazine, Modern Maturity

3200 East Carson Street
Lakewood, CA 90712
310-446-2277

Healthy Older People
National Health Information Center

Center for health information for diseases such as AIDS, cancer, diabetes, etc., substance abuse, and insurance, including Medicare and Medicaid

800-336-4797

Life Extension Foundation

Information available on life extension and funding in gerontology

800-327-6110

National Council on Aging

Information line capable of answering questions/problems of the elderly

800-424-9046

National Elder Care Institute on Health Promotion

Database clearinghouse of information—health promotion topics—programs, videos, brochures

601 E Street NW
Fifth Floor
Washington, DC 20049
202-434-2200
202-434-6474

National Institute on Aging Information Center

Clearinghouse of information for the elderly

PO Box 8057
MSC Suburban, MO 20898-8057
800-222-2225
301-589-3014

Emergency Services

Medic Alert Foundation US

Service provides an "ID tag" engraved with personal medical facts, as well as a 24-hour emergency response center which can release additional personal medical details

800-432-5378
209-669-2477

Environmental

Environmental Protection Agency
National Pesticide Information Clearinghouse

Information available on specific chemicals; environmental, ecological effects and household cleanup/disposal questions

800-858-7378
800-743-3091 – Texas only

Environmental Protection Agency
Safe Drinking Hotline

Information about regulations at the federal level that apply to drinking water systems

800-426-4791

Environmental Protection Agency Public Information Center

Referral service and general, non-technical information on a variety of EPA programs

PM–211B
401 M Street SW
Washington, DC 20460

202-260-2080
202-260-6257

Toxic Substances Control Act Assistance Information Service

Document distribution; answers questions, both technical and non-technical, about pollution prevention, lead, etc.

401 M Street SW
Washington, DC 20024
202-554-0515
202-554-5603 (fax)

Epilepsy

Epilepsy Foundation of America

Counseling, group sessions, Social Security information, information on housing for disabled

800-EFA-1000
212-967-2930

Eyesight

National Eye Care Project Hotline

National outreach program designed to provide medical eye disease care to disadvantaged seniors

800-222-EYES

National Eye Institute

Information on eye diseases or disorders, biomedical research

Building 31, Room 6A32
9000 Rockville Pike
Bethesda, MD 20892
301-496-5248

Family Health

American Association for Marriage & Family Therapy

Sends out information and list of therapists in your zip code area

800-374-AMFT

Family Life Information Services/Exchange

Substance abuse prevention, funds raised to work with policemen on prevention

PO Box 37299
Washington, DC 20013-7299
800-526-9038
301-585-6636

Lifeplan Family Caring Network, Inc.

Underwriters of long term care insurance, research and development on long term care, information and referrals

800-525-7279

Fitness & Sports Medicine

AFAA (Aerobics and Fitness Association of America)

Certification in aerobics and fitness instruction

15250 Ventura Boulevard, Suite 310
Sherman Oaks, CA 91403
800-446-2322 – California only
800-225-2322 – Rest of the Nation
818-905-0040

American Running & Fitness Association

Information and literature available on exercise and physical fitness, especially running, and safety

800-776-ARFA

Aquatic Exercise Association

Referral source for aquatic therapy and fitness

PO Box 497
Port Washington, WI 53074
813-486-8600

Presidents Council on Physical Fitness and Sports

Set up programs to promote nationwide health and fitness

701 Pennsylvania Avenue NW, Suite 250
Washington, DC 20004
202-272-3430
202-504-2064 (fax)

YMCA of the USA

Health and physical education/fitness information

101 North Wacker Drive
Chicago, IL 60606
800-USA-YMCA
312-977-0031

Gay & Lesbian Services

Lavender Health Services

Support services for gay, lesbian and bisexual individuals and their families; free literature available listing help lines and other support groups, counseling and related services

Office of Gay & Lesbian Health Concerns
New York City Department of Health
New York, NY 10013
212-788-4310

Lesbian & Gay Community Services Center (The Center)

Offers information, literature, support groups, referral services and counseling for gay, lesbian and bisexual individuals

208 West 13th Street
New York, NY 10011
212-620-7310

Handicapped

Jobs Accommodation Network

Information available on accommodations in the workplace for handicapped workers

800-526-7234 (M-F, 8:30 AM-4:30 PM EST)
800-526-4698 (WV only)

National Clearinghouse on Postsecondary Education for the Handicapped

General questions answered and informational literature available

800-544-3284

National Easter Seal Society

Over 160 affiliates offering speech and language rehabilitation, occupational therapy, treating of development/learning disabilities

800-221-6827

National Organization of the Disabled
Special Projects

Information on the disabled, including the American Disabilities Act

800-248-ABLE

National Center for Youth with Disabilities

Informational resource center focusing on adolescents with disabilities

800-333-6293

Hanson's Disease

Hanson's Disease
American Leprosy Missions

Information available on Hanson's disease and related topics as well as information on fund raising for clinics to treat leprosy

800-543-3131

Head Injury

National Head Injury Foundation

Information and resource specialists available to assist in answering questions and/or mailing out literature on head injury

800-444-NHIF

The New York State Head Injury Family Helpline

Offers chapters, support groups, resources and materials for traumatic head injury patients and their families

800-228-8201

Headache

National Headache Foundation

Information available on headache causes and treatments, state member physician listing available

800-843-2256

Heart Disease

American Heart Association

Materials available on health maintenance, nutrition, dieting, smoking, research and community programs; local chapters in each county

National Center
7272 Greenville Avenue
Dallas, TX 75231
800-AHA-USA1

National Heart, Lung, And Blood Institute Education Programs Information Center

Publications available relating to cardiovascular diseases, asthma education, cholesterol and other health problems; makes referrals to other organizations

PO Box 30105
Bethesda, MD 20824-0105
301-251-1222

Home Care and Hospice

American Health Care Association

Information on long-term care, how to choose a hospice program or assisted living residence, information on Medicaid and how to pay for nursing home care are a few topics on which consumers may obtain information

1201 L Street, NW
Washington, DC 20005
202-842-4444

Hospice Education Institute–Hospice Link

A phone-in service which maintains a list of hospice programs across the country and will refer a caller to a program in his/her area. Books available on hospice care

190 Westbrook Road
Essex, CT 06426
800-331-1620

National League for Nursing–Community Health Accreditation Program (CHAPs)

Accredits home care agencies throughout the nation. Call for accreditation status

350 Hudson Street
New York, NY 10014
212-989-9393
800-669-1656

Foundation for Hospice and Home Care

Consumer guide entitled, "All About Hospice Care" is available on how to choose a home care agency. This agency also certifies home care aides and accredits some home care agencies

519 C Street, NE
Washington, DC
202-547-6586

National Association for Home Care

Publication entitled, "How to Choose a Home Health Agency" is available by sending a self-addressed, stamped envelope to the following address:

519 C Street, NE
Washington, DC
202-547-7424

National Hospice Organization

Local referrals to hospices in area, answers general information questions and sends out literature

1901 North Moore Street, Suite 901
Arlington, VA 22209
703-243-5900
800-658-8898

Huntington's Disease

Huntington's Disease Society of America

Information and literature available on Huntington's Disease offering assistance to the afflicted and their families

800-345-4372
212-242-1968 – New York City only

Impotence

Impotence Information Center

Information specialists available to answer questions and mail out literature pertaining to impotence

800-843-4315

Incontinence

Simon Foundation

Sends out general information packet on incontinence and will refer out to other organizations to answer questions

800-23-SIMON

Infertility

The American Fertility Society

Pamphlets and brochures available as well as referrals to area physicians

205-978-5000

Injury

National Head Injury Foundation

Information related to injuries of the head. Literature available.

202-296-6443

Kidney Disease

American Kidney Fund

Assists in funding the treatment of indigent dialysis patients, comprehensive educational programs provided, research grants, community projects

800-638-8299

800-492-8361 – Maryland only

Kidney Stones

Brochures available on the treatment of kidney stones

800-333-3032

National Kidney and Urologic Diseases Information Clearinghouse

Information on kidney disease, urinary tract infections and related topics

PO Box NKUDIC
9000 Rockville PIke
Bethesda, MD 20892
301-654-4415
301-770-5164 (fax)

National Kidney Foundation

Research organization: Information specialists available to answer questions and distribute information on diseases of the kidney and/or related problems

800-622-9010

Lead Poisoning

National Lead Information Center Hotline

Information to help prevent lead poisoning; makes referrals to state and local offices for individuals to receive further information

800-LEADFYI

Liver Disease

American Liver Foundation

Information available on liver disease and related problems

800-223-0179
201-256-2550 – New Jersey only

Living Will

Choice in Dying

Provides counseling on choices and information on living wills

200 Varick Street
New York, NY 10014
212-366-5540
800-989-WILL

Lou Gehrig's Disease

ALS Associates

Provides information and education on Lou Gehrig's Disease and refers families to local support groups

800-782-4747

Lung Disease

American Lung Association

Informational number for lung disease, smoking cessation, and general health

Director of Communications
1740 Broadway
New York, NY 10019-4374
212-315-8700

Cystic Fibrosis Foundation

Free information and literature available on Cystic Fibrosis including referrals to local support groups and treatment centers

800-344-4823
301-951-4422

National Jewish Center for Immunology and Respiratory Medicine

Literature available and nurses on staff to answer questions

800-222-5864
303-355-5864 – Colorado only

The American Lung Association of New York

Answers questions, operates a referral service and will mail literature at callers' request

212-889-3370

Lupus

Lupus foundation of America

Twenty-four hour information and referrals to local chapters available

800-558-0121
301-670-9292 – Maryland only

Lupus Hotline
Lupus Foundation of America

Free information packet available and further information available through toll call to business office

800-558-0121
301-670-9292 (business office)

Lyme Disease

American Lyme Disease Foundation

Information available on Lyme Disease prevention as well as how to recognize the symptoms and seek medical assistance

Mill Pond Offices
293 Route 100
Somers, NY 10589
800-876-LYME
914-277-6970

Medical Alert

Medical Alert Foundation US

Service provides an "ID tag" engraved with personal medical facts, as well as a 24-hour emergency response center which can release additional personal medical details.

800-432-5378
209-669-2477

Lifeline Systems

"Lifeline" information on systems which enable direct lines from the elderly or handicapped to hospitals

800-451-0525
617-923-4141 – Massachusetts, Hawaii and Alaska only

Mental Health

American Mental Health Fund
National Mental Health Association

Information available on clinical depression and mental illness; directory of local mental health association and referral services; contributions accepted

800-433-5959

The Door

Adolescent health center providing legal services, counseling, education, unity programs

121 Avenue of the Americas
New York, NY 10013
212-941-9090

National Alliance for the Mentally Ill

Information available on support groups for the mentally ill

800-950-6264

National Institute of Mental Health

Free publications and referrals available for questions

5600 Fishers Lane, Room 15C05
Rockville, MD 20857
301-443-4513

National Mental Health Association

Information available on mental health/illness and local support groups, informational clearinghouses, etc.

800-969-6642
703-684-7722 – Virginia only

The National Resource Center on Homelessness and Mental Illness

Information source; periodic bulletin on research, funding opportunities, and programming issues on homelessness and mental illness

262 Delaware Avenue
Delmar, NY 12054
800-444-7415

Suicide Prevention Resources (not a hotline)

Educational organization and programs, training programs, counseling services, resource directory

347 East 61st Street, Room 1RE
New York, NY 10021
212-750-8410

Mental Retardation

American Association on Mental Retardation

General information available on mental retardation

800-424-3688

Multiple Sclerosis

National Multiple Sclerosis Society

Questions answered by phone and general information literature available on research, neurologists and MS centers; local chapters in each county

1-800-344-4867

Neurological Disorders

Tourette Syndrome Association

Forty-eight chapters of support group services, referrals, research and education for families of those afflicted

800-237-0717

Nutrition Information

American Dietetic Association Consumer Nutrition Hotline

Information on nutrition available as well as referrals to local nutrition counselors

800-366-1655 (10:00 AM– 5:00 PM CST)

Food and Nutrition Information Center

Lending services, food and nutrition publications, general information, information specialists available to answer questions

Department of Agriculture
National Agricultural Library, Room 304
10301 Baltimore Boulevard
Bellsville, MD 20705-2351
301-504-5719
301-504-5472 (fax)

Human Nutrition Information Service

Information available on nutrition, consumption, dietary guidance and nutrition education

US Department of Agriculture
6505 Belcrest Road
Hyattsville, MD 20782
301-436-7725
301-436-5078 (electronic bulletin board)

National Center for Nutrition & Dietetics, Nutrition Hotline
American Dietetic Association

Registered dietitians available to answer questions on nutrition information, weight maintenance, food guide, food labeling, and refers out to local registered dietitians

800-366-1655

Organ Donor Programs

The Living Bank

Organ donor registry for those interested in donating organs after death

800-528-2971
800-GIFT-4-NY (New York regional office)

United Network for Organ Sharing

For those interested in registering to receive an organ under the guidance of one's personal physician

800-243-6667

Organ Donor Hotline
North American Transplant Coordinator Organization

Information available on organ donation and organ transplant

800-24-DONOR

Osteoporosis

National Osteoporosis Foundation

General information available on osteoporosis

2100 M Street, NW, Suite 602 B
Washington, DC 20037
800-223-9994

Parenting

A Way Out

Parental hotline: counselors available for parents who have abducted their children

800-A-WAY-OUT

Mothers without Custody

Information available by mail on custody and/or visitation rights

PO Box 27418
Houston, TX 77227-7418
800-457-6962

National Maternal and Child Health Clearinghouse

Literature and information specialists available to answer questions

8201 Greensboro Drive, Suite 600
McLean, VA 22102
703-821-8955, ext. 254 or 265
703-821-2098 (fax)

Parents Anonymous

Counseling available for parents who are/have been involved in child abuse and/or abusive relationships

800-352-0386 – California only

Parents Without Partners

Information available on local support groups for single parents

800-637-7974
301-588-9356 – Maryland only

Parkinson's Disease

American Parkinson's Disease Association

Counseling and referrals made in addition to providing literature on treatment

800-223-2732

National Parkinson's Foundation

Questions answered; research, adult day care, literature, and referrals are available

800-327-4545
800-433-7022 – Florida only
305-547-6666 – Miami area only

Parkinson's Educational Program

Publications available and referrals made to support groups

800-344-7872 – to receive literature on Parkinson's Disease
714-250-2975 – to speak with staff member
514-640-0218 – California only

Pesticides

National Pesticides Telecommunications Network

Information available on various pesticides

800-858-7378

Plastic/Reconstructive Surgery

American Academy of Facial Plastic and Reconstructive Surgeons

General information and lists of local surgeons available

800-332-3223

American Society of Plastic and Reconstructive Surgeons

Surgical procedure information available as well as referrals and verification of credentials

800-635-0635

Cosmetic Surgery Information Services

Brochures on various procedures and referrals to local doctors available

800-221-9808

Facial Plastic and Reconstructive Surgery Information Service

Brochures on different types of facial plastic surgery and referrals to board-certified plastic surgeons

800-332-FACE
800-523-FACE – Canada only

Pregnancy Services

ASPO/Lamaze

Provides information on Lamaze technique and refers out to local clinics

800-368-4404

American Academy of Husband-Coached Childbirth

Free information on the Bradley method available as well as lists of instructors in your local area

800-422-4784

Birthright/Abortion Alternative

Confidential pregnancy counseling to pregnant girls and provides maternity, baby clothes and support services including medical and financial referrals

800-848-5683

Edna Gladney Center Pregnancy Hotline

Counselors available to discuss options when pregnant, especially adoption; residential services available for women putting babies up for adoption

800-433-2922
800-926-3304 – Texas only

International Childbirth Education Association

Pregnancy, childbirth and infant care information available

800-624-4934

La Leche League International

Information available on breast feeding

800-525-3243 (9:00 AM–3:00 PM CST)

Planned Parenthood

Clinic offering education, counseling and medical care to women faced with pregnancy and other medical problems

800-248-7797 – White Plains, NY only
212-274-7200 – Manhattan only

Primary Care Information

National Clearinghouse for Primary Care Information

Publications and/or consultants available for general information

8201 Greensboro Drive, Suite 600
McLean, VA 22102
703-821-8955, ext. 245
703-821-2098 (fax)

Public Policy

Agency for Health Care Policy and Research Clearinghouse

Publications available dealing with health care issues and policies

PO Box 8547
Silver Spring, MD 20907-8547
800-358-9295
301-495-3453
301-589-3014 (fax)

Rare Disorders

National Organization for Rare Disorders (NORD)

The services through this organization include reports on rare diseases and symptoms, a networking program for those afflicted by the same diseases, and a listing of other organizations to contact. Annual membership for NORD is $25. NORD prints newsletters three times a year

PO Box 8923
New Fairfield, CT 06812
800-999-6673
203-746-6518
203-746-6519

Rehabilitation

American International Health and Rehabilitation Service

Information available on health care and rehabilitative medicine

800-362-1822
800-548-9719

National Rehabilitation Information Clearinghouse

Information on disabilities and technical products for people with disabilities

8455 Colesville Road, Suite 935
Silver Spring, MD 20910
800-346-2742
301-588-9284
301-587-1967 (fax)

Retinitis Pigmentosa

National Retinitis Pigmentosa Foundation

Answers questions and has available information on the latest developments in RP

Baltimore, MD
800-683-5555

Reye's Syndrome

National Reye's Syndrome Foundation

Information on symptoms of Reye's syndrome and on treatment and support networks

800-233-7393
800-231-7393 – Ohio only

Schizophrenia

American Schizophrenia Association

Focusing on all types of mental disorders, primarily schizophrenia, publishes journals and bulletins on quarterly basis for purchase, refers out to other physicians

510-841-8361

Sexual Addiction

Sexual Addiction Treatment and Training Institute

Information and treatment available

1 Patchin Place
New York, NY 10011
212-366-1490

Sexual Compulsives Anonymous

Counselors available to answer questions, send literature, and refer to support groups

212-439-1123

Sexually Transmitted Diseases

STD National Hotline

Confidentially provides free information about STDs and provides referrals for diagnosis and treatment

800-227-8922

Sickle Diseases

Sickle Cell Disease Association of America

Provides referral lines and referrals to local chapters, educational materials, counseling

Culver City, CA
800-421-8453

Skin Disorders

American Society for Dermatologic Surgery

Provides information on surgical procedures related to skin damage from the sun, disease, or aging

800-441-2737
9 AM–5 PM (Central Time) Monday–Friday

Smoking & Health

Office on Smoking and Health

Information and literature available on smoking cessation and general health problems related to smoking

Public Information Branch
Park Building, Room 1-18
5600 Fishers Lane
Rockville, MD 20857
301-443-1575

Office on Smoking and Health Center for Chronic Disease Prevention and Health Promotion

Literature and/or publications available

Centers for Disease Control
MS K-50
1600 Clifton Road NE
Atlanta, GA 30333
404-488-5705
404-488-5767 (fax)

Social Security And Insurance

Insurance Information Institute

Offers general information on life, health, home and auto insurance

800-942-4242

Social Security Administration

Information on Social Security claims and general information concerning eligibility

Washington, DC
800-772-1213 – Social Security Hot Line

Spinal Cord Injury

American Paralysis Association

Data available on spinal cord injury and other central nervous system disorders

800-225-0292

National Spinal Cord Injury Association

Information available for patients and families on organizations, agencies, and local support group services

Woburn, MA
800-962-9629

Spinal Cord Injury National Hotline

Information available on spinal cord injuries and related problems

800-526-3456

Stroke

Stroke Connection of the American Heart Association

Information and consulting available as well as referrals to local support groups

7272 Greenville Avenue
Dallas, TX 75231-4596
800-553-6321

National Stroke Association

Information and support groups available for stroke victims and their families

800-787-6537

Stuttering

National Center for Stuttering
Stuttering Hotline

Answers questions, provides literature and offers support groups

800-221-2483
212-532-1460 – New York City only

Substance Abuse

ADAPT: Association for Drug Abuse Prevention and Treatment

Refers out for substance abuse of any kind and HIV+

552 Southern Boulevard
Bronx, NY 10455
718-665-5421

Alcohol and Drug Dependence Helpline

Information on alcohol and/or drug abuse available 24 hours a day

800-821-4357

Alcoholics Anonymous - NY ENTOL Group

Meetings and fellowship sharing in support groups

212-647-1680

AL-ANON Family Groups

Self-help group for families of alcohol and drug abusers

PO Box 862 Midtown Station
New York, NY 10018
800-344-2666

American Council on Alcoholism

Information on alcoholism prevention, programs, counseling and referrals to treatment programs

5024 Campbell Boulevard, Suite H
Baltimore, MD 21236
800-527-5344
410-889-0100 – Baltimore only

The Center for Substance Abuse Treatment National Drug Hotline

Counseling, referral service, general information on substance abuse and addiction

800-662-4357

Families Anonymous, Inc.

Provides information and counseling to families and/or others related to a substance abuser or someone with behavioral problems

PO Box 528
Van Nuys, CA 91408
818-989-7841

Just Say No Foundation

Drug prevention, educational clubs (peer pressure and awareness), discussion and programs

800-258-2766

Mothers Against Drunk Driving (MADD)

General information, statistics of alcohol related fatalities, victim information, support groups and counseling

800-438-6233

Narcotics Anonymous

Twelve step, self-help group of addicts working with addicts to recover from addiction

World Services, Inc.
PO Box 9999
Van Nuys, CA 91409
818-780-3951

National Clearinghouse for Alcohol and Drug Information

Information and referrals to callers regarding alcohol and drug treatment programs

PO Box 2345
Rockville, MD 20852
800-729-6686

National Cocaine Hotline

Twenty-four hour hotline offering information, literature and referrals to assist substance abusers

800-COC-AINE

National Council on Alcoholism & Drug Dependence, Inc.

Affiliated offices and phone numbers given for those suffering from drug addiction and/or alcohol dependence

800-NCA-CALL

Center for Substance Abuse Treatment

Literature, information and referrals available to assist those in need of counseling and/or rehabilitation

800-662-HELP

New Life (Women for Sobriety)

Provides help and assistance to women alcoholics

800-333-1606

Office of Substance Abuse Prevention's National Clearinghouse for Alcohol And Drug Information

Information available on all aspects of substance abuse

PO Box 2345
Rockville, MD 20847-2345
800-729-6686
301-468-2600
800-487-4889 (TT)
301-468-6433 (fax)

Target National Resource

Provides information on healthy lifestyle, primarily for high school athletic /activity participants

800-366-6667

Sudden Infant Death Syndrome

SIDS National Headquarters

Information available on how to prevent SIDS; referrals available

800-638-7437 (24-hour hotline)

Surgery Service

National Second Opinion Surgical Program
Department of Health and Human Services

Information available on receiving second opinions through Medicare

800-638-6833
800-492-6603 – Maryland only

Traffic Safety

National Highway Traffic Safety Administration (NHTSA)

Report auto safety problems; safety literature available including information on recalled automobiles and child car seats as well as tire information

800-424-9393 (hotline)
202-366-0123 in DC (hotline)

Travel

International Association for Medical Assistance to Travelers

716-754-4883

International SOS Assistance

215-244-1500
800-523-8930

Urologic Disorders

American Foundation for Urologic Disease

Information on urologic disorders, prostate cancer and incontinence, infertility, urinary tract infections; refers out to cancer survivors; support groups

800-242-2383
410-727-2908 – Baltimore only

Veterans Services

Eastern Paralyzed Veterans Association

Educational classes offered ranging from architecture to wheelchair repair; sports and recreational programs and hospital liaisons (counseling) offered to veterans with a spinal cord injury

75-20 Astoria Boulevard
Jackson Heights, NY 11370-1178
718-803-EPVA

Victim Services

Hate Crimes National Hotline (US Dept. of Justice)

To report knowledge of and/or victimization due to any crime linked to intolerance

Constitution Avenue & 10th Street, NW
Washington, DC 20530
202-514-3204

Weight Loss

Take off Pounds Sensibly (TOPS)

4575 South 5th Street
Milwaukee, WI 53207
800-932-8677

Women's Health

American College of Obstetricians and Gynecologists

Provides information and educational material on health issues related to obstetrics and gynecology

409 12th Street, SW
Washington, DC 20024
800-673-8444
202-638-5777 – District of Columbia only

Breast Implant Information Service

Provides information on the status of clinical studies being conducted on silocone breast implants

Food & Drug Administration
PO Box 1802
Rockville, MD 20704-1802
800-532-4440
800-688-6167 TTY
9 A.M. to 5 P.M. EST, Monday–Friday

Johnson & Johnson, Inc. Personnal Products Consumer Response Center

Provides information on women's health concerns, including TSS (Toxic Shock Syndrome)

New Brunswick, NJ 08901
800-526-3967

Women's Sports Foundation

Information on women and sports, physical fitness and sports medicine

800-227-3988

Note: These numbers and addresses change frequently and without notice. You may have to make a number of calls to track down a source or organization.

Medical Records Appendix M

There are very good reasons for making certain you obtain your medical records, starting with the fact that you will be a more informed health consumer and better able to participate in medical decisions affecting your life. You may avoid repeat testing, thus saving money, time, and unnecessary exposure. You will provide your physician with a more accurate and comprehensive medical history, which will result in better care. By keeping your medical records you will also be able to ensure their accuracy.

In most states, patients have a legal right to their medical records. In fact, the new terminology is "patient record," not "medical records." Traditionally, there has been resistance from the medical community, which feared that such access might be harmful to patients or prompt some of them to treat themselves. The legal release of medical records has shown these fears to be largely groundless.

Although the hospital or doctor may charge you a reasonable price for photocopying, you can rarely be denied the records. In some states, for example, access may be denied only if the information can reasonably be expected to cause harm to the patient or others, or the material consists of personal notes and observations. If access to patient records is denied, you have a right to appeal that decision, usually through your state health department.

Doctors

There are three types of records patients should obtain and hold for safekeeping and to share with physicians: hospital records, physician records, and records from the Medical Information Bureau, a shared service of insurance companies. Among the specific medical records you should obtain are:

Current medical status

History of present illness

Physical exam results

Test results

Past medical history
i.e., hospitalizations, surgeries, allergies, drug reactions, medications

Social history
i.e., marital status, diet, sexual history

Reports of consultants and conferring physicians

Family history
i.e., family illnesses and causes of death

Review of systems
i.e., the baseline data of each system of the body

Medical Information Bureau (MIB)

Hospitals

Medical records come from two primary sources: your doctor and any hospital in which you have been a patient. Hospital records will include information from a variety of sources in addition to your physician, including nursing staff, pharmacy, and insurer. It will begin with an admissions work-up and conclude with a discharge summary. Reporting on the reason for your admission, treatment and length of stay, your hospital records could include X-rays, radiologist reports, pathologist reports, blood and urine tests, daily progress charts and notes, including blood pressure, pulse rate, nursing notes, physician notes, and medications. The discharge summary is the most important document and includes a description of your condition at time of discharge and future medication and treatment recommendations.

Medical Information Bureau

The Medical Information Bureau (MIB) is a data base that provides information to some 750 insurance companies nationwide. When you applied for most health, life, or disability insurance policies, you undoubtedly signed a waiver permitting your insurance company to share medical records with other companies.

MIB was founded by insurers to protect them from fraud and omission. If an insurance applicant has a condition significant to health or longevity, member companies are required to send a brief, coded report to MIB. Medical conditions are reported by using one or more of about 210 codes. There are also five limited codes for reporting nonmedical information that might affect insurability. These include:

1. adverse driving record
2. participation in hazardous sports
3. aviation (pilot or regular member)
4. known or suggested association with criminal activity or related violence
5. possible overinsurance

An example of an MIB record is printed in their fact sheet, appearing as follows:

SMITH, ELLIOT A.	
040C34	VA
MGR	
A31MY84	300GZN-
(341ZF)	200ZF
Y06OC85	347SZN
Y09DC86	900#X#

It is important that the information on file at MIB is accurate. Your insurability may be in question if it is not. To obtain your records, call the MIB at 617-426-3660 or write to:

PO Box 105
Essex Station
Boston, MA 02112

If you find the record in error, ask the MIB about its procedures for correcting it.

Sources of Medical Information Appendix N

Many services are available to assist consumers in researching personal medical questions and/or problems. Although not meant to replace a doctor's diagnosis, the medical literature searches and software packages listed below may serve as a guide in the search for a greater understanding of a disease or a search for alternative cures and treatments. Some of the software packages also track health histories, office visits, and the finances involved in family health management.

Medical Information Services: Searches medical literature for the public

AIC Services

313-996-5553

- For profit
- Labor charge of $50/hour plus computer charges
- Average cost $150-400

Health ACCESS

914-232-6628

- For profit
- Mini report includes an overview of disease and listing of abstracts for $75
- Full report includes an overview, summaries, full articles, a listing of clinical trials, and a list of relevant organizations concerned with the subject for $150 to $200

The Health Resource

501-329-5272

- For profit
- $150 for Medline Source
- $225 for Medline search plus PDQ cancer topics
- $85 for mini reports

The Michigan Information Transfer Source (MITS)

313-763-5060
FAX 313-936-3630

- Non-profit
- Labor charge of $60/hour plus computer and phone charges
- Average cost $200-500

Medical Information Service

800-999-1999
415-326-6000

- Non-profit
- $89 provides all citations published in last 2-3 years on Medline
- PDQ & Directory to Organizations

Planetree

415-923-3680

- Non-profit
- $25 for 25 titles of articles without summaries
- $75 for maximum of 40 citations
- $100 for above plus PDQ information

Somatech

203-364-1221

- For profit
- Labor charge of $50/hour plus computer and phone charges
- Average cost $150-250
- A multi-disciplinary staff, including MDs and PhDs, provides interpretations of data. Information is accompanied by a report offering recommendations and alternative treatments.

Medical Information Line

900-230-4800
($1.75 per minute. Topics average five minutes)

Using Your Personal Computer (Software)

Creative Multimedia Corp.

503-241-4351
CD-ROM

- Articles on common medical issues by columnist Dr. Allan Bruckheim

Healthdesk

800-578-5767

- Records family history
- Tracks physician fees
- Tracks dates of vaccinations

Stedman's Plus/Data Cal

800-336-5988 (for book)

- Medical and pharmaceutical terms
- Dictionary for spell checking medical and legal documents.
- List of trade and generic drug names

Mayo Clinic Family Health Book/Interactive Ventures

800-692-4000
CD-ROM

- First Aid
- Nutrition
- Disease
- Health System

Med$ure: Your Health Insurance Manager!

Time Solutions
800-552-3302
203-459-0303

- File and track medical claims
- Policy comparisons
- Tax savings from your benefits
- Family immunization and health history
- Record book
- Glossary of medical insurance terms

Personal Physician/Familycare Software
800-426-8426
- Quizzes about symptoms
- Suggests treatments
- Comes with real stethoscope

Healthsoft/Great Bear Technology
800-795-4325
- Calculates personal health risks based on personal regimens (eating, exercising, etc.)

On-Line Through Commercial Computer Services

Dialog
800-3DIALOG
- Medline costs $36/hour, plus $0.07 per citation

BRS
800-955-0906
- $33/hour plus $0.15 per citation and $12-33/hour for communication charges

LEXIS/NEXIS
800-346-9759
- $6/minimum to run a check on a doctor's name and background; run can last from 5 to 15 minutes. There is a $.05 charge per line, for printing, averaging $2.50 per charge.

On-Line through National Library of Medicine
- Medline costs $16.50/hour on off hours and $22/hour during prime time, plus $0.01 per printed line

ORBIT
800-45-ORBIT
Compuserve
- Medline is not available through ORBIT

DATASTAR

800-221-7754

- Medline costs $36.10/hour, plus $.11 per citation and $11/hour for telecommunication charges.

Sources of Information and Assistance for Health-Care Consumers

Special Resources

The following list describes a group of organizations and agencies that offer information and assistance to consumers and/or to health care professionals. Some are specific services (e.g., Centers for Disease Control and Prevention Fax Information Service for International Travelers).

All of the professional organizations listed are important leaders in shaping health care policy in the nation. Consumers should be aware of these organizations, their function and purpose, and how they can be contacted.

National Organizations & Agencies

Agency for Health Care Policy & Research

(AHCPR) A component of Public Health Service (PAS). Its goals are to promote effective, appropriate, high-quality health care; increase access to care; and improve health services. It operates a national publication clearinghouse.

AHCPR Publications Clearinghouse
PO Box 8547
Silver Springs, MD 20907
800-358-9295

American Ambulance Association

800-523-4447

To check on accreditation of an ambulance service or to obtain general information on EMS services.

American Board of Medical Specialties

To ascertain whether or not a physician is board-certified; offers free publications.

1007 Church Street, Suite 404
Evanston, IL 60201-5913
708-491-9091

American College of Radiology

Educational materials are for member radiologists but some are available to the public.

703-648-8900
703-648-8792

American Hospital Association

Trade association which lobbies and researches for hospitals—not a consumer help line.

1 North Franklin Street
Chicago, IL 60606
312-422-3000

American Medical Association

Referral information; check on physicians' credentials; information and literature available.

312-464-5000

Centers for Disease Control and Prevention (CDC)

Fax Information Service for International Travelers

This service provides free, immediate faxed reports on disease risk and prevention and disease outbreaks in various parts of the world.
Fax: 404-639-1733

Commission on Accreditation of Ambulance Services

The accreditation body for all ambulance services which can tell you the status of the accreditation of all/any ambulance services.

PO Box 619911
Dallas, TX 75261-9911
214-580-2829

Federal Information Center Program

Referral service for various federal agencies. The GSA also offers a number of free or low cost publications, many dealing with health care, to consumers.

General Services Administration
Seventh and D Streets SW
Washington, DC 20407
301-722-9098

Food and Drug Administration

Tests and approves drugs and devices; investigates reports of food contamination; approves mammography labs.

301-443-1544
800-358-9295 (mammography)

Health Care Financing Administration (HCFA)

Oversee financing and administration of Medicaid and Medicare.

200 Independence Avenue, SW
Room 314 G
Washington, DC 20201
202-690-6726

Health Outcomes Institute

Offers information on the development and use of tools and techniques for measuring the effectiveness of health care.

2001 Killebrew Drive
Bloomington, MN 55425
612-858-9188

Medicare and Medicaid

Department of Health and Human Services
Inspector General's Hot Line
800-368-5779
800-638-3986 - Maryland only

National Center for Health Statistics

General information on nationwide health statistics available.

6525 Belcrest Road, Room 1064
Hyattsville, MD 20782
301-436-6154

National League for Nursing (& CHAP)

Accrediting body for schools of nursing which also publishes books, tapes and tests for nurses, health care professionals, and consumers.

350 Hudson Street
New York, NY 10014
212-989-9393

National Network of Libraries of Medicine

Reference materials available for research into medicine and/or disease and health care.

800-338-RMLS

National Practitioner's Data Bank

Maintains information on disciplinary actions taken against doctors. All state medical licensing boards, hospitals, HMOs and health clinics must check with the Bank prior to issuing a license to a doctor. The information, however, is not available to the general public.

Rockville, MD
301-443-2300

ODPHP'S National Health Information Center
(Office of Disease Prevention and Health Promotion)

Informational pamphlets available on diseases (e.g., AIDS, cancer, and asthma) as well as Medicare, Medicaid, and drug abuse.

PO Box 1133
Washington, DC 20013-1133
800-336-4797
301-565-5112 (fax)

Office of Minority Health Resource Center

Bilingual operators available to send out free information on health topics of special interest to minority groups.

1010 Wayne Avenue, Suite 300
Silver Spring, MD 20910
800-444-6472

People's Medical Society

A wide variety of medical and health care literature available to consumers on any and all health care topics.

800-624-8773

Health Care Planning: Living Wills and Health Care Agents Appendix O

The thought of death is not a comforting one to most people and planning for the last stages of life is not a task most of us approach enthusiastically. Only about 15 percent of Americans have made any advanced planning for end-of-life care, despite the fact that about 70 percent said they would decide against life-sustaining measures if they found themselves incompetent with a poor prognosis. The lack of an effective plan for this stage of life not only affects the quality of our last days but has tremendous financial implications. The cost of uncontrolled care in a loved one's last days can sometimes wipe out a family's financial resources. Nationally, about 28 percent of annual health spending is utilized by the six percent of Medicare enrollees who die in that year. With more than 30 million people, or 12 percent of the population, aged 65 and older, this is a significant health, financial, and ethical issue in our society.

There are two steps an individual should take in order to plan in advance for a potentially prolonged death. The two most necessary steps are preparing a living will and appointing a health care proxy or agent. These are best done in conjunction, although each can be done individually.

A living will is a document that spells out, as precisely as possible, the kind of medical treatment you desire to sustain life when you are unable, because of illness or injury, to provide direction.

The appointment of a health care proxy or agent, through a durable power of attorney, is designed to empower someone else to make decisions concerning your health care and, particularly, life-extending efforts, if you are incapable of doing so. Although a living will can describe your wishes concerning the use of life-support measures such as mechanical breathing and artificial feeding, it cannot offer guidance for a decision such as whether you should be placed in a nursing home or whether a surgical or medical solution is the best approach. The health care proxy, with a health care durable power of attorney, may make those decisions.

It is best to prepare these documents with medical, legal, and religious advice and the documents must be signed voluntarily. They are also reversible by the signer at any time. Copies of living wills and health care proxies can be obtained from:

Choice In Dying
200 Varick Street, 10th Floor, Suite 1001
New York, NY 10014
(212) 366-5540

Health Care Proxy

I, ____

hereby appoint ______________________________
(name, address & telephone number)

as my health care agent to make any and all health care decisions for me, except to the extent that I state otherwise. This proxy shall take effect when and if I become unable to make my own health decisions.

Optional instructions: I direct my agent to make health decisions in accord with my wishes and limitations as stated below, or as he or she otherwise knows. (Attach additional pages if necessary)

____

____

(Unless your agent knows your wishes about artificial nutrition and hydration [feeding tubes], your agent will not be allowed to make decisions about artificial nutrition and hydration.)

Name of substitute or fill-in agent if the person I appoint is unable, unwilling or unavailable to act as my health care agent

____

Unless I revoke it, this proxy shall remain in effect indefinitely, or until the date or conditions stated below. This proxy shall expire (specific date or conditions, if desired):

____

Signature ________________________________

Address ________________________________

Date ________________________________

Statement by witnesses (must be 18 or older)

I declare that the person who signed this document is personally known to me and appears to be of sound mind and acting of his or her own free will. He or she signed (or asked another person to sign for him or her) this document in my presence.

Witness 1 ________________________________

Address ________________________________

Witness 2 ________________________________

Address ________________________________

Reading Materials of Interest Appendix P

An Unfinished Revolution: Women and Health Care in America, *Emily Friedman, Editor, United Hospital Fund, New York, 1994, 304 pp.*

Nineteen leading health care writers and scholars contributed to this book which traces the uneven progress women have made in reshaping the health care system, long regarded as a man's domain. From educational and professional victories to the still unresolved issues of gender bias and equity in health care services, the book offers valuable information and insights into present-day problems that women face as patients and providers in the health care system.

The Best Doctors in America *by Steven Naifeh and Gregory White Smith, Woodward and White, Inc., Aiken, 1992, 712 pp.*

This book lists over 3,700 doctors, nationwide, by specialty, subspecialty, and particular expertise of techniques. It is similar in purpose to the well-known Woodward and White publication which lists lawyers.

The Best Doctors in the U.S. *by John Pekkanen, USA Wideview Books, New York, 1980, 290 pp.*

Although somewhat dated, Pekkanen's book, first published in 1970, seems to be the first of the genre. He not only lists whom his research led him to conclude were the 500 best doctors in the country by specialty, but he describes the hospitals and health centers he believes to be the best for treating various diseases and health problems.

The Best in Medicine *by Herbert J. Dietrich, MD, and Virginia H. Biddle, Harmony Books, New York, 1990, 212 pp.*

This book outlines the authors' selection of the best medical centers and hospitals in the United States. The book is organized by disease entity or procedure, for example, cancer or organ transplants. This book would be useful to someone engaged in a search for medical assistance, regardless of cost or geography.

The Best Medicine: How to Choose the Top Doctors, the Top Hospitals, and the Top Treatments *by Robert Arnot, MD, Addison-Wesley Publishing Company, Reading, 1992, 468 pp.*

Dr. Arnot lists doctors and hospitals across the nation that his research has led him to believe are the best in treatment of specific specialties or ailments. Included are chapters on heart, obstetrics and gynecology, orthopaedics and burn, as well as chronic diseases including AIDS, arthritis, cancer, and depression (this is a partial listing). This is a very useful book for someone searching for assistance when distance and cost is not a factor.

The Columbia-Presbyterian College of Physicians and Surgeons Complete Guide to Early Childcare *Nicholas Cunningham, MD, Medical Editor, Crown Publishers, 1990, 514 pp.*

This volume calls itself the book that tells you everything you need to know about your child up to the age of five. Everything you need to know includes not only medical problems, behavioral challenges, and growth patterns, but also how to make the most of your relationship with a most important person in your child's life: the pediatrician.

The Complete Guide to Living Wills *by Doron Weber, Bantum Books, New York, 158 pp.*

This useful work is a comprehensive overview of the intricacies of the planning and use of living wills and related issues.

The *Good Housekeeping* Illustrated Guide to Women's Health *Kathryn Cox, Medical Editor, Hearst Books, 1994, 380 pp.*

Published by the popular women's magazine, this volume offers comprehensive advice on health and health care issues of concern to contemporary women. Of special interest are sections on how to navigate the health care system, and how to stay healthy in the workplace.

Communicating With Your Doctor *by J. Alfred Jones, MD, and Gerald M. Phillips, Southern Illinois University, Carbondale and Edwardsville, 1988, 184 pp.*

Dr. Jones and Phillips review a variety of topics including selecting a doctor, the doctor-patient relationship, barriers to collaboration, and understanding how doctors function. It contains much useful information, but the organization of the book and the variety of subjects makes it necessary to read it in its entirety in order to obtain that which is useful.

Consumer's Guide to Hospitals, *Consumer's Checkbook, Washington DC, 1994, 224 pp.*

By the editors of Consumers' CHECKBOOK magazine, this guide is, primarily, an analysis of the death rates at 5,500 hospitals based on HCFA (Health Care Financing Administration) data. It also includes brief chapters on keeping costs down and learning about your particular case.

The Consumers Guide to Medical Lingo *by Charles B. Inlander and Paula Brisco, People's Medical Society, Allentown, 1992, 95 pp.*

A handy paperback that contains definitions and explanations of medical health care ranging from diagnostic tests to medications, as well as a listing of insurance terms.

The Consumers Legal Guide to Today's Health Care *by Stephen L. Isaacs, JD, and Ava C. Swartz, MPH, Houghton Mifflin Company, Boston, 1992, 384 pp.*

This book uses a legal perspective and framework to assist the consumer in navigating through the health care system. It includes chapters on patient's rights, health insurance, job related issues, long term care, Medicare, Medicaid and specific health problems such as abortion, reproductive technologies and AIDS.

Could Your Doctor Be Wrong? *by Jay A. Goldstein, MD, Pharos Books, New York, 1991, 247 pp.*

This book is a listing of diseases, symptoms and potential causes. It is written for the person who may feel their physician is incorrect in diagnosing or managing their problem.

Diagnosing Your Doctor: A Straightforward Guide to Asking the Right Questions and Getting the Health Care You Deserve *by Arthur R. Pell, PhD, DC Publishing, Minneapolis, 1991, 50 pp.*

Dr. Pell provides a useful overview of how to obtain good health care. The title, "Diagnosing Your Doctor," is not reflective of the total scope of the book which includes chapters on health insurance, HMOs, nursing homes and medical check ups.

How to Choose a Good Doctor *by George K. LeMaitre, Andover Publishing Group, Andover, 1979, 169 pp.*

This book is a good overview on selecting doctors. It includes chapters on avoiding surgery, over and under-doctoring, and getting the most out of your visit to your doctor.

How to Talk to Your Doctor: The Questions to Ask *by Janet M. Maurer, MD, Simon & Schuster, Inc., New York, 1986, 205 pp.*

Organized primarily on a question-explanation basis, this book is thorough in answering relevant questions on everything from common illnesses to medications; from understanding an illness to hospitalization. It also includes a glossary of medical terms including roots and prefixes and suffixes of complex medical terminology which help consumers better understand their illness and prescriptions.

150 Ways to Be a Savvy Medical Consumer *by Charles B. Inlander, the People's Medical Society, Allentown, 1992, 96 pp.*

This easy-to-read guide covers, in concise listings, everything from how to save money at the doctor's office to how to avoid costly billing errors. It instructs the reader on how to be knowledgeable about health care by listing simple tips on saving money without sacrificing sound medical care.

Patient Power *by John C. Goodman and Gerald L. Musgrove, Cato Institute, Washington DC, 1992, 673 pp.*

The subtitle to this book is "Solving America's Health Care Crises." Despite the somewhat misleading title, the book is an interesting read that analyzes much of what the authors see to be wrong with American health care today.

The People's Hospital Book *by Ronald Gots, MD, PhD, and Arthur Kaufman, MD, Crown Publishers, New York, 1978, 211 pp.*

Covering the selection of a hospital, analyzing physician care,and understanding procedures and equipment, this book informs and advises on how being a more informed health care consumer will make your hospital stay a better one. With a chapter on how to cut frustrations in emergency departments, this is a book for all—even for those who do not plan on a long hospital stay.

The Savvy Patient *by David R. Stutz and Bernard Feder and the Editors of Consumer Reports Books, The Consumers Union, Yonkers, 1990, 276 pp.*

One of many useful books and reports published by Consumers Union, this book describes how the patient can best interact with the medical system. It stresses the relationship between doctor and patient, particularly in terms of knowledge, authority and power. It also describes how patients can maintain stronger control over their medical care and treatment.

Second Opinion *by Isadore Rosenfeld, MD, Bantam Books, New York, 1987, 435 pp.*

Dr. Rosenfeld is a prolific medical writer. His work explores not only the general principles of using second opinions, but talks specifically about selected diseases and conditions, and tells when a second opinion may be useful or necessary.

The Silent World of Doctor and Patient *by Jay Katz, MD, The Free Press, a division of MacMillan Inc., New York, 1984, 263 pp.*

This book touches on all aspects of the doctor patient relationship, including trust, legal responsibilities, sharing authority, and the historical basis and evolution of this relationship. Although well written and very readable, it is probably a more extensive view than the layperson would want to take.

Source Book of Health Insurance Data, *Health Insurance Association of America, Washington, DC, 1992, 141 pp.*

Specific information, outlined in the form of text and graphs, is easy to understand. From the overview of the health insurance industry to facts and data on costs, resources, enrollment, and utilization, this book is full of statistics which may be of use to those researching hospitals and/or HMO enrollment.

Taking Charge of Your Medical Fate *by Lawrence C. Horowitz, MD, Random House, New York, 1988, 319 pp.*

Dr. Horowitz's book is divided into three sections. The first discusses why taking charge is critical to your health. He emphasizes hysterectomies, C-sections, cancer, heart disease, drugs, and tests to make his points, which include the variability of hospital quality. The second section discusses obstacles and briefly explores the roles and relationships of doctors and patients. The third section tells the reader how to take charge, which is primarily a discussion of how to use the health care system effectively.

10,289 Questionable Doctors *2 Vols. by Sidney Wolfe, MD, and Phyllis McCarthy, et al, Public Citizen, Washington, 1993.*

A complete list, by state, of physicians disciplined by the states or the federal government from 1986 through 1993. It gives the physician's personal and practice information, as well as outlines the offense and disciplinary action taken.

The Woman's Guide to Good Health *by Mary Gray, MD, and Florence Hazeltine, MD, et. al.,Consumer Reports Books, New York, 1991, 468 pp.*

Drs. Gray and Hazeltine, both trained in obstetrics and gynecology (Dr. Hazeltine in reproductive endocrinology as well) have written a very useful book for women interested in knowing more about the problems and issues that will affect them directly. Among the topics explored are female sexuality, the breasts, the reproductive system, menstruation, infertility, birth control, cancer and menopause.

REPORTS

National Directory of Adult Day Care Centers
Health Resources and American Business Publishing
908-681-1133

Consumers' Guide to Hospitals
Consumers' Checkbook
733 15th Street, Suite 820
Washington, DC 20005
202-347-7283

AHA Guide to the Health Care Field
American Hospital Association
1 North Franklin Street
Chicago, IL 60606
312-422-3000

Medicare Hospital Information Report
Separate volumes listing the mortality information for every hospital on a state-by-state basis are available by writing:
Government Printing Office
Superintendent of Documents
Washington, DC 20402-9320

Mortality Report for Coronary Artery By-Pass Surgery
An analysis conducted in New York State for mortality during or immediately following coronary by-pass surgery is available by writing:
Cardiac
Box 2000
New York State Department of Health
Albany, NY 12220

INDEX

A

B

C

D

E

F

G

H

I

M

N

O

P

T

U

W

Editor: Sue Berkman
Publications Coordinator: Amy Beth Czebatol
Design: Harper & Case, Ltd.